TAI-CHI CHUAN

in Theory and Practice

TAI-CHI CHUAN
in Theory and Practice

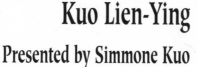

Kuo Lien-Ying
Presented by Simmone Kuo

North Atlantic Books
Berkeley, California

Tai-Chi Chuan in Theory and Practice

Published by North Atlantic Books
P.O. Box 12327
Berkeley, California 94712
Cover art by Professor Yao You-Wei, Yang Zhin University, China
Cover and book design by Nancy Koerner
Printed in the United States of America

Tai-Chi Chuan in Theory and Practice is sponsored by the Society for the Study of Native Arts and Sciences, a nonprofit educational corporation whose goals are to develop an educational and crosscultural perspective linking various scientific, social, and artistic fields; to nurture a holistic view of arts, sciences, humanities, and healing; and to publish and distribute literature on the relationship of mind, body, and nature.

Library of Congress Cataloging-in-Publication Data

Kuo, Lien Ying.
    Tai-chi chuan in theory and practice / Lien-Ying Kuo : edited by
Simmone Kuo.
        p.   cm.
    ISBN 1-55643-298-4 (alk. paper)
    1. T'ai chi ch'uan. I. Kuo, Simmone. II. Title.
GV504.K855 1999
613.7'148--dc21   98-38444
                                              CIP

2   3   4   5   6   7   /   04   03   02   01   00

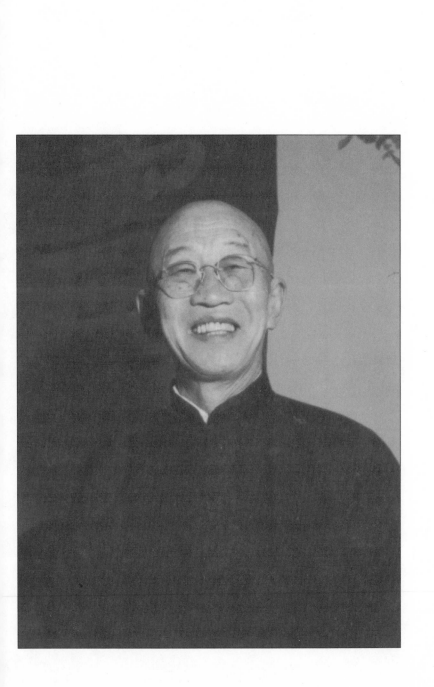

Table of Contents

郭連蔭太極拳譜

于右任

Dedication

This is the third edition of Sifu Kuo Lien-Ying's English version of *Tai-Chi Chuan in Theory and Practice*. The first edition appeared before his "journey to the west" while Master Kuo was still living in China; the second edition came out in 1966, soon after his immigration to the United States.

Master Kuo studied and practiced the martial arts throughout his long life; and, of these, his favorite was Tai-Chi Chuan. Sifu was a dedicated student of Sifu Wang Chiao-Yu. He remembered and respected his vow to transmit Tai-Chi Chuan as he had received it from Grand Master Wang. Every morning before practicing he recited the 13 Tai-Chi stances from the mnemonic poem in 144 characters which hung from his wall.* Knowing that this was important to him, I also follow his method and want to share it with the public. Sifu's experience, knowledge and perseverance are a legacy to be treasured.

I have appended some basic material on Tai-Chi philosophy and the *I-Ching* to Sifu's original text, in hopes that modern students of Tai-Chi Chuan will be inspired to reflect upon the historical and philosophical sources of the art. In addition, I have included a small selection of some of Sifu's favorite literature to inspire further reading.

Since the Lien-Ying Tai-Chi Chuan Academy opened in August of 1965, we have been blessed to receive and teach thousands of students. Late in his life, in 1980, Sifu was happy to see the dream he had carried

See page 17, "A Mnemonic of Thirteen Tai-Chi Chuan Movements" for English translation of this text.

to the west come true—Tai-Chi Chuan being studied and taught as physical education in the Department of Kinesiology at San Francisco State University, and thus being integrated into American culture as a whole.

It is a joy for me to see the treasured art of Tai-Chi Chuan flourishing throughout the modern world. My hope is that the method embodied in this book will guide its development in the best of all possible directions.

Simu Kuo
1998, Year of the Tiger

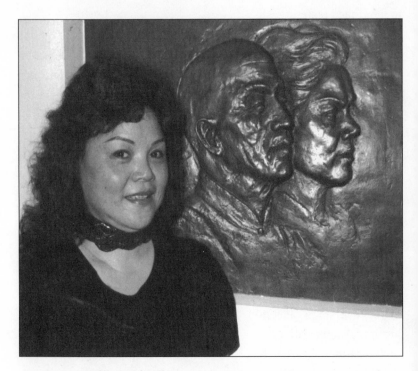

Simmone Kuo with Kuo family appreciation plaque at Chinese-Americans for Affirmative Action, San Francisco

以心行氣神達多方
若鶴之躍猶龍之翔
蓮陰大師正
溥儒

when the mind
is still
in the heart

vital energy flows
and the spirit expands
permeating all creation

like ten thousand birds
soaring and wheeling
in the form of a great dragon[1]

yin and yang
soft and hard
balance

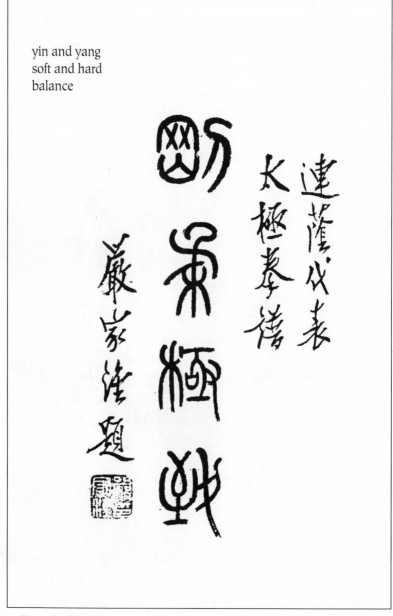

Calligraphy by Yen Jia-Gan, vice-president, Taipei, Taiwan Province, 1960.

Foreword

Some years ago I wandered into Professor Kuo Lien-Ying's Tai-Chi Chuan studio in San Francisco. At the time, I did not comprehend the nature of the journey I was about to embark upon. Yet in some uncanny way I felt compelled to begin the practice of Tai-Chi Chuan under the guidance of Professor Kuo and his wife. Perhaps it was the profound sense of peace and tranquillity emanating from the students that enticed me to study Tai-Chi Chuan. At the time I was a psychologist, a profession demanding an intense emotional and intellectual response, requiring no involvement whatsoever of the physical side of one's being. It is ironic that psychotherapy's design to enhance levels of health and well-being rarely mentions the importance of physical exercise in treatment programs. The daily practice of Tai-Chi Chuan was soon to teach me that to attain balance in life—which in the ancient Chinese medical treatise, *The Yellow Emperor's Classic of Internal Medicine*, is synonymous with good health—one must partake of exercises designed to enhance both the mind and the body. To place undue emphasis on one dimension at the expense of the other is foolhardy, leading to conditions of ill health and disease, as is the case in contemporary Western society with its exaggerated concern with the mind. The physical activity expressed in the Tai-Chi Chuan form is a "Yang" phenomenon associated with improved circulation, muscle tonus, and respiration, while thinking is essentially a "Yin" phenomenon, passive and non-assertive in nature. It is as a result of excessive thinking and ruminative behavior that all manner of pathological conditions arise. The activity inherent in the Tai-Chi Chuan form is a proven remedy for such maladies.

Though I was good with words and skilled in my profession, having undergone years of therapy, I was nonetheless unhappy, and lacking vitality. Something seemed to be missing in my life. That something, I was soon to learn, was the expression of "intrinsic energy," a latent source of vitality that could be awakened by the form. Mrs. Kuo explained the benefits of Tai-Chi Chuan and chided me that my body would not benefit from her verbal description, only by daily practice. The tendency of the Tai-Chi Chuan Master to say little about his or her art has its origins in Taoist thought, where verbal rhetoric is considered to be of lesser importance to the health of the organism than the silent, concentrated, physical expression of the form. The *I-Ching*, the most ancient compendium of Chinese wisdom, reflects upon the deceptive use of language in Hexagram 31, line 6, as follows:

Six at the top means: one's influence shows itself in the jaws, cheeks, and tongue.[2]

The explanation of these lines is as follows:

The most superficial way of trying to influence others is through talk that has nothing real behind it. The influence produced by such mere tongue wagging must necessarily remain insignificant.

In Hexagram 37 of the *I-Ching*, entitled "The Family," the correct use of words is alluded to as follows:

The superior man is said to have substance in his words, and if words and conduct are not in accord they will have no effect.

In Tai-Chi Chuan, skill is manifest in the form, not in one's description of how proficient he is. One might say the form speaks for itself. My teacher's tendency to de-emphasize rhetoric in favor of vital action stands in direct contrast to contemporary Western man's intellectual approach to phenomena, where words and verbal gymnastics are meant to mystify, and creative physical activity is viewed as a lesser vehicle of expression. Our preoccupation with the faculties of the mind and minimal concern with motor functioning accounts for the prevalent of psychosomatic disorders in our culture. Numerous times I've observed Master Kuo walk among his students mimicking with his lips their too-lengthy verbal discourses, pointing out to them through his mime-like gestures how much more important it is to practice Tai-Chi Chuan than to discuss it. The development of a daily practice routine is essential if one is to really commune with the essence of the form. By performing the movements each morning one learns to apply himself more diligently and creatively to all of life's undertakings. Gradually any tendency toward laziness and lethargy is replaced by a renewed sense of vigor and increased energy output.

The development of a mature disciplined character capable of withstanding frustration was seen by Carl Jung as one goal of the therapeutic process. Jung and his student, Marie Von Franz, developed the concept of the *"puer aeternus,"* the "eternal child," to describe that being who is forever living in fantasy, preferring inaction and lassitude to worldly demands. Though the *puer* is ready at a moment's notice to work himself twenty-four hours at a stretch on an exciting, lofty project, he has no patience whatsoever for anything resembling an ordinary way of life. Jung saw the cure for the *puer's* weakness in "work," in activity demanding a practical response that would gradually develop this immature aspect of his personality. Von Franz comments on the psychology of the *puer* as follows:

> When he [the *puer*] has to take something seriously, either in the outer or inner world, he makes a few poor attempts and then impatiently gives up. My experience is that it does not matter, if you analyze a man of the type, whether you force him to take the outer or the inner world seriously; that is really

unimportant . . . The important thing is that he should stick something out . . . do something through, but the great danger, or the neurotic problem, is that the *puer*, or the man caught in this problem, just puts it in a box and shuts the lid on it in a gesture of impatience . . . and they always do it at the moment when things become difficult.[3]

For those of us possessing some degree of the *puer's* nature, Tai-Chi Chuan poses an excellent remedy. Through daily practice of the form we develop a positive mental outlook, while our body is energized to take on even the most boring of activities from a new perspective. By persevering and refining each move we learn what it is to develop patience.

In my first lesson Mrs. Kuo familiarized me with the six warm-up exercises that serve as a sound foundation for performing the sixty-four movements that make up the form. These exercises are designed to enhance flexibility, strengthen the musculature, tendons and bones, and improve circulation. Wholistic medicine recognizes the human need to expel accumulated gases and noxious wastes from the organism. The warm-up exercises facilitate this process in a gentle yet dynamic manner. Tai-Chi Chuan adepts claim that "long tendons lead to a long life." The warm-up stretches are designed to increase flexibility while strengthening the organism down to its deepest level, "the marrow of the bones." Each of the stretches presents the student with a difficult task, and only diligent and regular practice will lead to attainment of the goal. At the time I began practice my body was tense, rigid, and uncoordinated. My teacher, on the other hand, could perform the stretches in a relaxed manner. I watched as Mrs. Kuo placed her chin to her toe from a forward bending position.

Apparently this was the most difficult of the warm-ups and had to be attained if one were to reap the full psychological and physical benefits of the Tai-Chi Chuan practice. Over the years I've heard it said that before the Tai-Chi Chuan form was taught to Professor Kuo in China, he first had to achieve this difficult stretch. Westerners on the other hand might not have the patience to persevere at this task unless they were given the rudiments of the Tai-Chi Chuan form while they were whittling away at the distance between chin and toe. So a compromise was reached and they were taught the moves even before they could perform "chin to toe." The gradual attainment of this goal has provided me with numerous insights into the structure and function of my anatomical parts as well as psychological insights into various aspects of my personality pertaining to patience and pain thresholds. One experiences a certain amount of discomfort and pain during the execution of the stretch as different parts of the body respond. During certain periods plateaus are reached. Further progress is temporarily halted, no matter how forcefully one strives towards the goal. At such times one immediately gets in touch with any tendency towards impatience and bullheadedness. When the body says "no" and the mind says "yes," a battle ensues which only a "yielding" to gentleness can remedy. The principle of "yielding" is firmly embedded in Taoist philosophy, and expressed in the Tai-Chi Chuan form not as an intellectual abstraction but as a physical reality from the inside of the body out.

Experiences such as the above affect the student at all levels and can't help but generalize to his everyday life. One is forced to remember in times of crisis that just as the "chin to toe" exercise cannot be attained by indiscriminate use of force applied to one's own body, such force applied to an outside adversary or conflicted situation will also prove futile. Here one is reminded of Hexagram 33 in the *I-Ching*, "Retreat," whose psychology of conflict resolution is as follows:

> . . . it is through retreat that success is achieved . . . retreat is not to be confused with flight. Flight means saving oneself under any circumstances, whereas retreat is a sign of strength.

The psychotherapeutic corollary of the "yielding" principle expressed philosophically in Taoism and physically in Tai-Chi Chuan is seen in Victor Frankl, M.D.'s logotherapy with its technique of "paradoxical intention." Instead of conducting a lengthy study into the motivational determinants directing his patient's dysfunctional behavior, Frankl encourages them to practice their symptoms. The obsessional who asks a never-ending stream of questions of himself and others is asked to spend more time engaging in such behavior than he is already doing. The pitifully shy, anxious individual is asked to visualize all the people in the room he is about to enter looking only at him. By repeatedly practicing these behaviors in fantasy and/or in action patients are freed from their compelling influence. By flowing with the behavior rather than opposing it, peace and tranquillity are attained. Frankl writes:

> This treatment consists of a reversal of the patient's attitude, inasmuch as his fear is replaced by a paradoxical wish. In other words, the wind is taken out of the sails of the phobia. This brings about a change of attitude toward the phobia. According to logotherapeutic teaching, the pathogenesis in phobias and obsessive-compulsive neuroses is partially due to the increase of anxieties, obsessions, and compulsions that is caused by the attempt to avoid anxieties or fight obsessions and compulsions. A phobic person usually tries to avoid the situation in which his anxiety arises, while the obsessive-compulsive tries to suppress and thus to fight his threatening ideas. In either case the result is a strengthening of the symptom. Conversely, if we succeed in bringing the patient to the point where he ceases to flee from or to fight his symptoms, but, on the contrary, even exaggerates them, then we may observe that the symptoms diminish and that the patient is no longer haunted by them.[4]

The Tai-Chi Chuan form taught by the Kuos is a beautiful sequence of meaningful movements coordinated into a synchronized flow of energy. One's physical health and sense of well-being are enhanced from the first moment's practice, while balance, poise, and the essence of spirit as expressed in the hands, take years to perfect. Performance of the movements over and over again leaves one feeling calm and relaxed, in accord with nature. No matter what calamities befall the student, the Tai-Chi Chuan practice is unimpaired and remains resilient in response to the aging process. Tai-Chi Chuan is both natural remedy and preventative medicine for much of what assails him. In today's chaotic times people often reach outside themselves for a panacea to their physical and emotional dilemmas. This tendency to look outside oneself to resolve problems is eschewed in the Chinese medical treatises and is referred to specifically in Hexagram 25 of the *I-Ching*, entitled "Innocence," as follows:

> Use no medicine in an illness incurred through no fault of your own. It will pass of itself.

The attitude alluded to here suggests that we take responsibility for our level of health and well-being, and not place our minds and bodies in the hands of the pharmaceutical industry.

In his book *Medical Nemesis*, Ivan Illich states that "the new burden of disease of the last fifteen years is itself the result of medical intervention in favor of people who are or who might become sick." It is doctor-made, or "iatrogenic." Illich cites statistics that illustrate the consequences to society of becoming overly dependent on medications and physicians. He states that "every 24 to 30 hours from 50 to 80% of adults in the U.S. swallow a medically prescribed drug, and that such drugs are addictive. In some patients antibiotics alter the normal bacterial flora and induce a superinfection permitting more resistant organisms to proliferate and invade the host. Other drugs contribute to the breeding of drug-resistant strains of bacteria." Illich summarizes his position with the following statement:

> A professional and physician-based health care system tends to mystify and to expropriate the power of the individual to heal himself and to shape his or her environment.[5]

Exercise may prove to be a partial solution to this dilemma, a means by which Americans can assume responsibility for their health and well-being.

The psychiatry and medicine of the future could benefit from the inclusion of Tai-Chi Chuan in any exercise program designed to restore health, improve self-esteem, and buoy one's spirit, for as Professor Kuo Lien-Ying states:

> The end purpose of these exercises is to prolong life, and to endow it with the youth of eternal spring.

Richard Vogel, Ph.D.

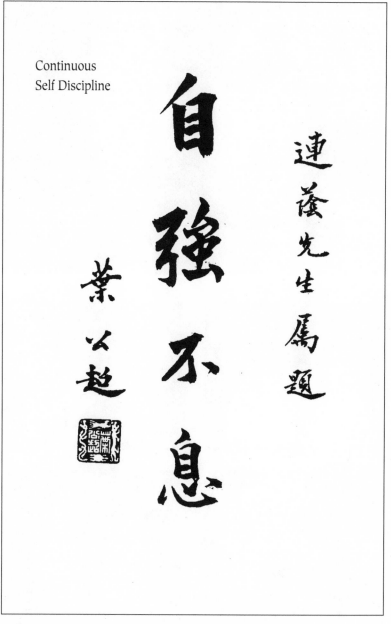

Continuous
Self Discipline

Calligraphy by Yie Gong-Chow, Taipei, Taiwan Province, 1960.

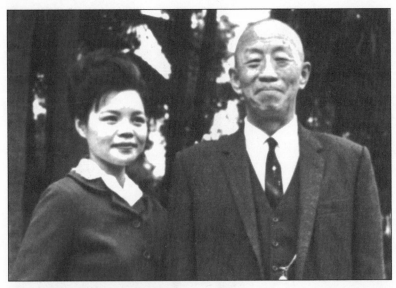

Taipei, 1966

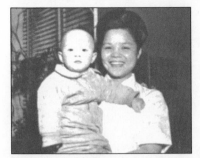
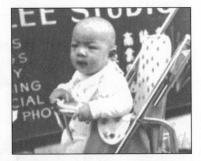

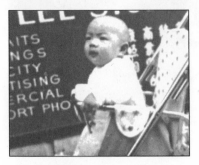
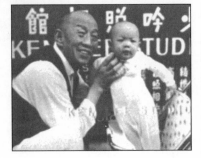

Kuo family outing, San Francisco, 1967

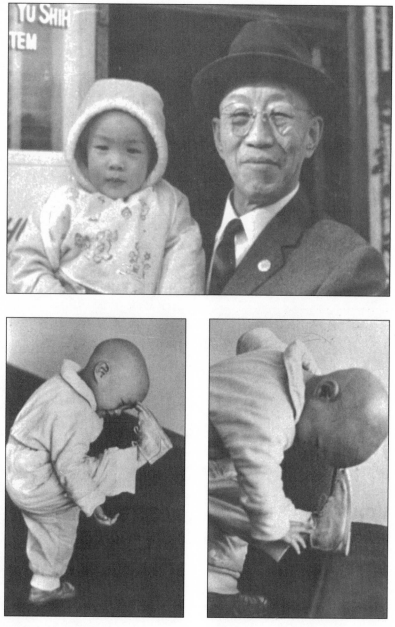

Father and Son

CHAPTER I

Discoursing on Tai-Chi Chuan

太極論

一舉動周身俱要輕靈，尤須貫串，氣宜鼓盪，神宜內斂，無使有缺陷處，無使有凸凹處，無使有斷續處，其根在於腳，發於腿，主宰於腰，形於手指，由腳而腿而腰，總須完整一氣，前進後退得機得勢，如不得機得勢處，身便散亂。其病必於腰腿求之。上下左右前後皆然，凡此皆是意，不在外面，有上即有下，有前即有後，有左即有右，如意欲向上，即欲下意，若將物掀起，而加以挫之之意，斯其根自斷，乃壞之速而無疑。

虛實宜分清楚，一處有一次虛實，處處總此一虛實周身節節貫串，無令絲毫間斷耳。

In any single movement of whatever sort, the whole body must move lightly, nimbly, and in coordination. The *chi** should be active as the propellant power behind all movements and the spirit should be gathered internally so that there will be no defects, nor uneven distribution, nor any discontinuity anywhere. The exercise has its root in the feet, is controlled by the waist and expressed by the fingers. The movement from feet upward through legs to the waist should always be fully coordinated. Seize the opportunity and size the situation in stepping forward or backward, otherwise the bodily movement will be confused. (By "opportunity" and "situation" we mean the kind of dynamic situation conducive to situations advantageous to yourself.) When confusion of movements occurs (that is, when different parts of the body move or remain without unified purpose), the cause is to be found in the waist or the legs. This test applies to movements in any direction. Nevertheless, the prime mover is the mind, not anything outside.

Everything is relative: the upper to the lower, the front to the back, the right to the left. If you intend to spring upward, bend downward first. You mean to raise a thing, but what you are doing may be actually pressing it down, so hard that the thing itself may be crushed. This happens whenever you violate a principle of the Tai-Chi philosophy.

The distribution of blankness and substantives should be clearly distinguished. This distribution can be found everywhere. Since such a distribution is found in each place, it forms a connected system throughout the whole body without any discontinuity.

---

*Chi *is the flux of energy or vitality including but not limited to the breath.*

CHAPTER 2

Key to Understanding the Thirteen (Tai-Chi Chuan) Movements

●

十三勢行工心解

以心行氣，務令沉着，乃能收歛入骨，以氣運身，務令順遂，乃能便利從心，精神能提得起，則無遲重之虞，所謂頂頭懸也。意氣須換得靈，乃有圓活之趣，所謂變動虛實也。發勁須沈着鬆淨，專重一方，立身須中正安舒，支掌八面，行氣如九曲珠，無微不利，氣遍身軀之謂運動，勁如百練剛，何堅不摧，形如攫兔之鶻，神如捕鼠之貓，靜如山岳，動似江河，蓄勁如開弓，發勁如放箭，曲中求直，蓄而後發，力由脊發，步隨身換，收卽是放，斷而復連，往復須有摺疊，進退須有轉換，極柔軟然後堅硬，能呼吸然後能靈活，氣以直奔而無害，動以曲蓄而有餘。心爲令，氣爲旗，腰爲纛，先求開展，後學緊湊，乃可臻於縝密矣！

又曰：先在心，後在身腹，鬆氣歛入骨，神舒體靜，刻刻在心，切記一動無有不動，一靜無有不靜，牽動往來，氣貼背歛入脊骨，內固精神，外示安逸，邁步如貓行，動勁如抽絲，全神意在精神，不在氣，氣在則滯，有氣者無力，無氣者純剛，氣若車輪，腰如車軸之謂也。

Be calm and steady in steering the *chi* with the mind, so that it can be absorbed and stored in the bones. Go easy and be natural in activating the body with the *chi*, so that it will coordinate with your mental command. When the spirit is fully aroused, there will be no fear of tardiness or clumsiness of movement. That is the meaning of holding up the head as if suspended from above. The change of aiming and breathing should be nimble enough to benefit itself from accommodating to the continually arising and changing situation. This is the meaning of transposition from one stance to another and the distribution of blankness and entities in a given movement.

Let the exertion of strength be steady, relaxed, neatly dosed, and all beamed to one focus at a time. Keep the body erect and comfortably occupying a central position, so poised as to be able to handle oncoming impact from all sides. Circulate the *chi* like threading pearls that have serpentine bores. The least crevice must suffice for passage. When the *chi* has circulated all through the body, call it a round of exercise.

Develop your strength until it is as resilient as highly tempered steel to which nothing is invulnerable. Poise your body like a hawk ready to pounce upon a rabbit, and alert your spirit like a cat ready to surprise a mouse. Where there is no motion, let it be as inert as the immobility of a mountain; where there is, let it be as fluid and adaptable to circumstances as rivers are to gradients. Store up your energy like the bending of a bow, and release it like shooting the arrow. Thus we see how the tortuous begets the straightforward—the more the bow is bent, the straighter speeds the arrow. There can be no release of anything without first accumulating it.

Strength is developed from the vertebrae, while the feet adapt their positioning in little steps in accordance with the demands of the trunk. In short, (Tai-Chi in action is both relative and self-reversible), intake is output, and disparates add up to continuity.

The alternation of stances must be relieved with variation, e.g., the forward and backward steps should leave enough space for one to turn around. First of all, learn to be as pliable as possible, for only then can one become hard and strong. To be short of breath is to lose agility altogether, while knowing how to breathe at ease under all situations keeps one nimble and alert (the results of sufficient reserve energy). To avoid harm, let the *chi* have full nurture and enjoy unhindered straight runs; to assure yourself of reserve energy, let your movements be in curves only.

In comparison with a military system, the mind is the commander's order; the *chi* is the messenger's banner that transmits the order; and the waist is the ensign that directs detailed operation.

In patterning movements into integrated wholes, let the component motions and blanks be loosely spaced, and keep the tempo relaxed. Gradually tighten up the composition and raise its tempo to the required degree (while bearing in mind the need for reserve energy).

The exercise should have its most important emphasis fall on the mind, and the next important in the body and abdomen. Release the *chi* and let it penetrate like a sword into the bones. Always keep your spirit at ease and body in quietude. Always remember that all parts of the body must move in unison and coordination; or, alternatively, all rest in quietude. In alternating movements, concentrate the *chi* to areas near your back, so that it may be, so to speak, absorbed into the vertebrae. Strengthen your spirit internally while you remain visibly comfortable outward expressions. Make your steps supple like a cat's, and exude your energy as if drawing out a silk thread (neither too taut, nor too slack, with even pull all the time). The whole concentration of mind is, however, on the sprit, not on the *chi*. When the mind concentrates itself on the *chi*, it will obstruct movement. Consequently, where the *chi* accumulates by being dammed up (like water), no power will be released; conversely where the sluice gate of *chi* is thrown open, invincible power may be generated, power as strong and solid as steel. Still another comparison, the *chi* may be likened to the spokes and rim of a wheel, of which the waist is the axis.

CHAPTER 3

Wang Tsung-Yue on Tai-Chi Chuan

王宗岳老先生太極拳論，一名長拳，一名十三勢，太極者，無極而生陰陽之母也，動之則分，靜之則合，無過不及，隨曲就伸，人剛我柔，謂之走，我順人背，謂之粘，動急則急應，動緩則緩隨，雖變化萬端，而理為一貫，由著熟而漸悟，懂勁而階及神明，然非用力之久，不能豁然貫通焉，虛靈頂勁，氣沉丹田，不偏不倚，忽隱忽顯，左重則左虛，右重則右虛，仰之則彌高，俯之則彌深，進之則愈長，退之則愈短，一羽不能加，蠅蟲不能落，人不知我，我獨知人，英雄所向無敵，蓋皆由此而及也。斯技旁門甚多，雖勢有區別，概不外乎壯欺弱慢讓快耳，有力打無力，手慢讓手快，是皆先天自然之能，非關學力而為也。察四兩撥千斤之重，顯非力勝，觀耄耋能禦眾之形，快何能為，如平準活似車輪，偏沉則隨，雙重則滯，每見數年純功，不能運化者，率皆自為人制，雙重之病未悟耳，雖欲避此病者，須知陰陽，粘即是走，走即是粘，陰不離陽，陽不離陰，陰陽相濟，方為懂勁，懂勁後愈練愈精，彌時揣摩，漸至從心所欲，本是舍己從人，多悟舍近求遠，所謂「差之毫釐，謬之千里」。學者不可不詳辨焉，是為之論，此論句句切要在心，并無一字敷衍陪襯，非有夙慧不能悟也。先師不可妄傳，非獨擇人，亦恐枉費工夫耳。

Discussing Tai-Chi Chuan, an authority of old, Wang Tsung-Yue told us that the exercise is also called *Chang-Ch'uan* (long boxing) or simply the Thirteen Movements. Tai-Chi or the Absolute is the originator of two equal and opposite principles: the Yin and the Yang; that is, the feminine, conserving or replenishing principle, and the masculine, activating or spending principle. Whenever there is motion, they separate; whenever there is motionlessness, they recombine. On the basis of this theory, Tai-Chi Chuan never over-exerts or under-exerts; it makes straight motions of circuitous ones. When an opponent's hard impact is met with yielding, it is called *tsou* or evasion. To follow up a retreating enemy motion without losing touch with it is called *chan* or adherence. Fast enemy attack is responded to with fast motion, while slow enemy momentum is followed up with slow motion. Although there are myriads of variations, there is only one basic principle, which can only be divided and understood through its practice. When one understands what strength is, he will also understand the true spirit of the art. (It is comforting to know that) after prolonged practice, one will, one day, all of a sudden, come to a full enlightenment (of its meaning and rationale).

While practicing, take care to keep your head buoyed up with intangible spirit, and let the *chi* sink to the *tan-tien* (which is situated on the horizontal line from the navel to the spine, and which divides this line at the ratio of 3:7 from the former). The movements are executed without leaning to any one side. The basic principle is expressed sometimes with

13

real motion, sometimes without. When the weight of fighting falls on your left-hand side, buffer it with blankness; and likewise for the right-hand side. (The concept of Tai-Chi so dwarfs understanding that) the more you look up, the loftier it rises; the lower you stoop down to reach it, the deeper it sinks. The more you press forward, the longer it stretches before you; the more you retreat, the shorter the span to do it in. The addition of a feather will be felt for its weight, and it is so free-moving that a fly cannot alight on it without setting it in motion. Your opponent is at a loss to know what you are about, but you know exactly what he will do next. Heroes are invincible just because of that.

There are many misleading ways of teaching the art of boxing. Although differing from one another, they all share one common principle, and that is: the stronger in brute force necessarily overwhelms the weaker, and the more sluggish must perforce yield to the more nimble. The one with physical strength thrashes the weakling; the slow-moving hand seeks in vain to dodge the fast-moving. But these are only empirical formulae which cannot take the place of true knowledge based on philosophical research. It is quite obvious that preponderance of physical strength alone does not explain the toppling of one thousand pounds with a trigger force of merely four ounces. He is not relying on speed when an old man successfully defends himself against the simultaneous attacks of many youthful strong opponents. (Something more than arithmetic is involved.) Keep the body in sensitive poise, so that it turns smoothly like a well-oiled wheel. Avoid inclining to either side, for that makes the body tend to fall to that side. Likewise do not divide your weight on both sides; if you did, your whole movement would be impeded. It has often been the case that one who has practiced boxing for several years but who has not mastered the correct principle, is usually beaten by his opponent. His divided attention (resulting in bilateral weight distribution) is to blame. In order to know the right thing to do, one has to understand the principles of the Yin and Yang. Thus *chan* is tantamount to *tsou*, and vice versa. The principles of Yin and Yang are

inseparable from one another. It is through a knowledge of this conjuga-
tory relationship that one comes to understand the way of fully and
effectively utilizing energy. After gaining such a knowledge, the more one
practices the art of Tai-Chi Chuan, the more skillful one becomes.
Through a long period of practice with intelligence and understanding,
one will gradually execute the movements according to his free will, for
by then his free will automatically choose the right movement. However,
many a beginner has honestly meant to give up bias and follow expert
instructions, when actually he was neglecting what was close at hand in
order to look for what is afar. (Truth is inherent in the here-and-now, not
imposed upon it by any foreign agency.) Deviation at the center of just a
hair's-breadth leads to divergence of a thousand miles at the circumfer-
ence. This is a point that students must always keep in mind. Of course,
only a man of wisdom can understand this, and that is the reason why
the former masters did not want to teach just anyone Tai-Chi Chuan: the
masters preferred to have the right kind of students because they did not
like to waste time.

CHAPTER 4

A Mnemonic of Thirteen Tai-Chi Chuan Movements

太極十三勢歌

　　十三總勢莫輕視，命意源頭在腰隙，變轉虛實須留意，氣遍身軀不稍滯，靜中觸動動猶靜，因敵變化亦神奇，勢勢存心須用意，得來不覺費工夫，刻刻留心在腰間，腹內鬆淨氣騰然，尾閭中正神貫頂，滿身輕利頂頭懸，仔細留神向推求，屈伸開合聽自由，入門引路須口授，工夫無息法自修，若言體用何爲準，意氣君來骨肉臣，想推用意終何在，延年益壽不老春，歌兮歌兮百四十，字字眞切義無遺，若不向此推求去，枉費工夫貽歎息。

L et no one esteem lightly
the Thirteen Movements,

But bear in mind that your consciousness of them commences in the waist,

In performance, care must be exercised regarding your transposition from
one stance to another, the twists and turns in each movement, and the
distribution of blanks and substantives in a given movement,

While keeping the *chi* freely circulating throughout your whole body.

All changes and motions are conceived and touched off in the stillness of
absolute quietude,

Hence motion and action are kindred to rest and inaction, in other words,
ultimately indistinguishable from each other.

Likewise, the mystery of Tai-Chi Chuan is that

It is your opponent's movements that condition your own as adapted by
nature to his own undoing.

Remember to be mindful of every single move by trying to feel its meaning,

And you will eventually come into possession of the art's secrets without
conscious effort.

Rivet your attention, without even a moment's interruption, onto the waist
interval, and

Keep your abdomen free from tension due to food or impurities, so that

Your vitality flux *(chi)* may, as it were, boil and rise like steam.

Keep the lowest segments of your vertebrae central in relation to gravitation all the while, when

Your limbs and body are gyrating with effortless nimbleness, and your head is held up buoyant as if suspended from above.

Carefully observe and investigate and convince yourself that

Your way of bending or straightening, your closing-in or throwing-open should never be as you will them to be, but as Nature wills.

A novice will require verbal instruction during the initial stages.

But practice will steer its own course and bring about its own perfection.

As to the theory and practice, i.e., the constituents and functioning of Tai-Chi Chuan,

The spirit is sovereign and the body its servant,

The end purpose of these exercises is to prolong life and endow it with the youth of eternal spring.

Oh, sing! Oh, sing! sing this short song of 144 Chinese characters;

Commit every single word of it to memory without exception.

Enquiries and researches that deviate from this approach

Only waste time and leave behind regrets and sighings.

CHAPTER 5

The Name of Tai-Chi Chuan

●

太極拳十三勢

太極拳原名爲長拳，過去有人認爲長拳就是十三勢，因爲根據路來說，長拳勢長，在太極拳論中說："長拳者，如長江大海，滔滔不絕也."

十三勢的名稱來源是這樣的：根據舊說，十三勢是包括了五行八卦在內，五行是金，木，火，土，比喻太極拳的五種步法；八卦是乾，坤，坎，离，巽，震，兑，艮，比喻太極拳的八種手法.

現在我們這樣理解：太極拳有五種步法，即：前進，後退，左顧，右盼和中定.手的用法有八種，即：掤，履，擠，按，採，列，肘，靠，分配在八個方向：東，南，西，北，東北，西北，東南，西南.這八方與前者五步合稱十三勢，也就是十三種方法的意思，若誤認爲十三勢式就錯了.

現將十三勢圖如下：

十三勢
　　　　　五步---前進，後退，左顧，右盼，中定
　　　　　　　　（金，木，水，火，土）.

　　　　　八方
　　　　　　　　四正（東，南，西，北）---掤，履，擠，按
　　　　　　　　　　　（乾，坤，坎，离）
　　　　　　　　四隅（東北，西北，西南，東南）採，列，肘，靠（巽，震，兑，艮）

What is called Tai-Chi Chuan was known earlier as Chang-Chuan (Long Fist), a colloquial name deriving from the continuous, spacious, and rhythmic quality of movement. The oral tradition comments that Chang-Chuan is like the waves of the Yangtze River, flowing endlessly.

A more formal way of referring to the practice was Shi-San Tse (the Thirteen Movements). In this name the philosophical origins of the art are evident: the Thirteen being composed of the Five Elements (which correspond to the positions of orientation to the earth's surface) and the Eight Trigrams of the *I-Ching* (which correspond to the directions of orientation in space). (See charts and diagram below.)

太極拳步法
Tai-Chi Chuan Movements
These are represented in the "Wu Shing" (Five Elements)

金 = 進　Advance

木 = 退　Retreat

水 = 左顧　Shift to the Left

火 = 右盼　Shift to the Right

土 = 中定　Stable Equilibrium

The name Tai-Chi Chuan was created in order to give the practice of this art the most universal naming possible: Chuan means fist, hence martial art; while Tai-Chi refers to the principle of ongoing creation—through balancing the primordial yin and yang energies. According to traditional Chinese philosophy the Thirteen Movements emerge out of various blendings of yin and yang.

As applied to movement, the five positions on earth are taken by the five foot positions—forward, backward, to the left, to the right, in the middle; while the eight directions in space are the eight hand actions of pushing hands and Pa-Kua Tsang. Thus, the Thirteen Movements signify the ways in which foot and hand motions are integrated as they emanate from the body's center—thirteen methods of movement, rather than thirteen particular acts of movement.[6]

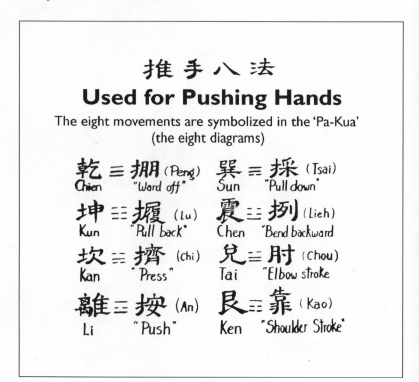

推手八法

Used for Pushing Hands

The eight movements are symbolized in the 'Pa-Kua'
(the eight diagrams)

乾 ☰ 掤 (Peng)
Chien   "Ward off"

巽 ☴ 採 (Tsai)
Sun   "Pull down"

坤 ☷ 攦 (Lu)
Kun   "Pull back"

震 ☳ 挒 (Lieh)
Chen   "Bend backward"

坎 ☵ 擠 (Chi)
Kan   "Press"

兌 ☱ 肘 (Chou)
Tai   "Elbow stroke"

離 ☲ 按 (An)
Li   "Push"

艮 ☶ 靠 (Kao)
Ken   "Shoulder Stroke"

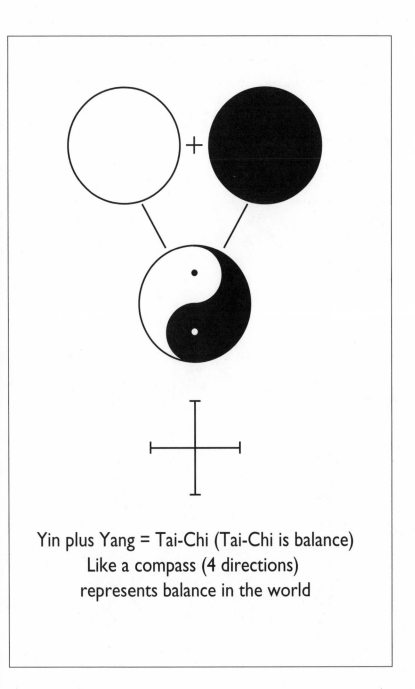

Yin plus Yang = Tai-Chi (Tai-Chi is balance)
Like a compass (4 directions)
represents balance in the world

CHAPTER 6

The Names of the Movements

●

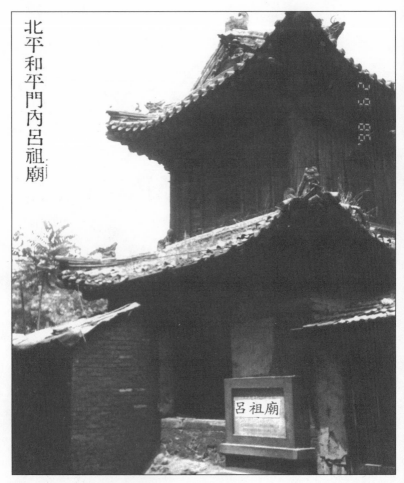

北平和平門內呂祖廟

呂祖廟

Li-Tzu Temple, Beijing.

Grand Master Wang Chiao-Yu taught Tai-Chi Chuan in the courtyard of Li-Tzu Temple until his death at the age of 104. Sifu Kuo Lien-Ying became his disciple in 1925; it was here that Sifu first studied and practiced.

Sifu always remembered and appreciated the purity of his teacher's transmission. Grand Master Wang passed on the original, traditional form of Tai-Chi Chuan with exactly 64 movements. Sifu followed his teacher's example and made no changes. In this way the form has remained connected to its true roots in the traditional philosophy of China, as first embodied in the 64 hexagrams of the ancient Book of Changes. (See Chapter 9, I-Ching and the Origins of Tai-Chi Philosophy.)

The names of the various movements of Tai-Chi Chuan are directly translated from the Chinese. Some of them describe the actual movements; others are names of applications of the movements; others are descriptive symbols taken from the natural world; still others are suggestive of imaginary creatures or events. The author would have standardized the names so that foreigners could easily understand the kind of movement meant by each name. However, he decided otherwise; for the original meanings might be lost and those acquainted with the original names might not be able to identify the new coinages. Fortunately, the names are of minor importance. They are retained for future revision. Even if some of the names are not comprehensible, practitioners can follow the given pictures so as to make the correct movements.

Please note, when more than one version of any movement occurs within the Tai-Chi Chuan form, that movement is pictured only once in the following sequence of photos. In this way we have preserved Sifu Kuo Lien-Ying's original layout.

29

CHAPTER 7

Illustration in Photos
of Tai-Chi Chuan

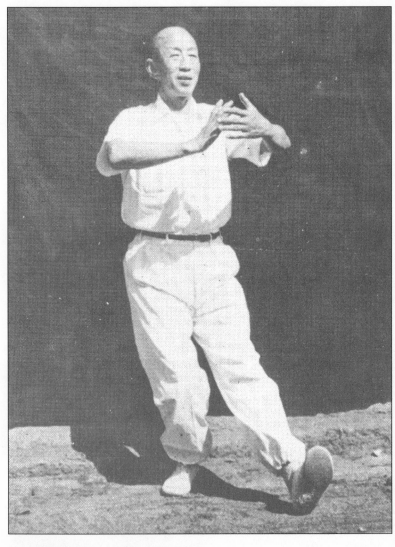

I. STRIKE PALM TO ASK BUDDHA

擊掌問佛　　Chi Chang Wen Fu

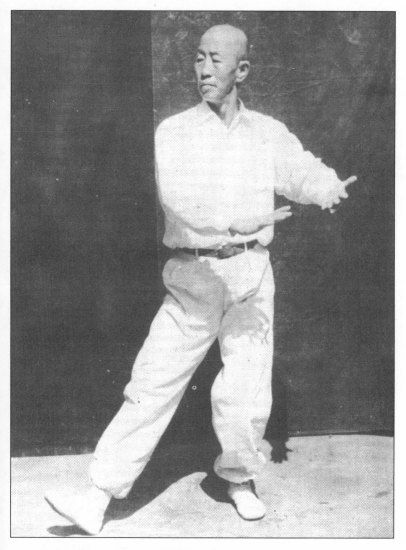

2. GRASP BIRD'S TAIL (LEFT STYLE)

攬雀尾（左式）　Lan Ch'iao Wei　(Tso Shih)

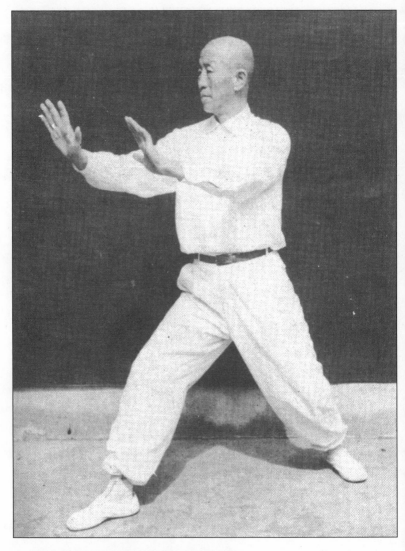

2. GRASP BIRD'S TAIL (RIGHT STYLE)

攬雀尾（右式） Lan Ch'iao Wei (Yu Shih)

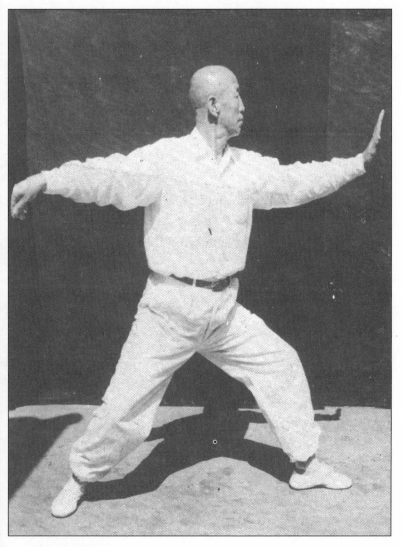

3. SINGLE WHIP

單鞭　　Tan Pien

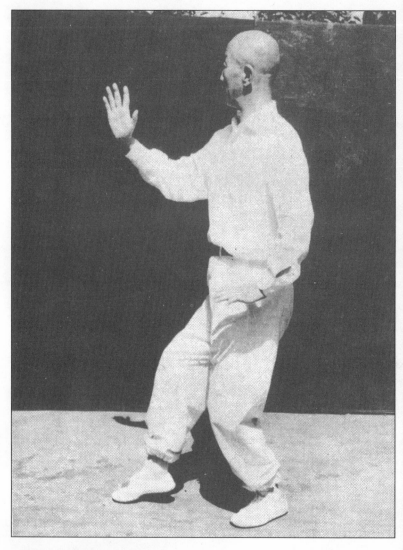

4. STORK SPREADS ITS WINGS

白鶴晾翅 Pai Hao Liang Ch'ih

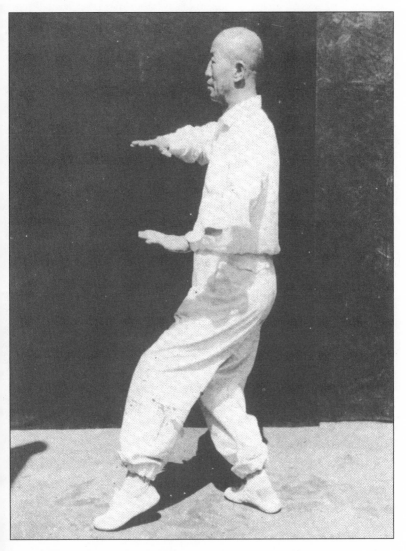

4. STORK SPREADS ITS WINGS

白鶴晾翅 Pai Hao Liang Ch'ih

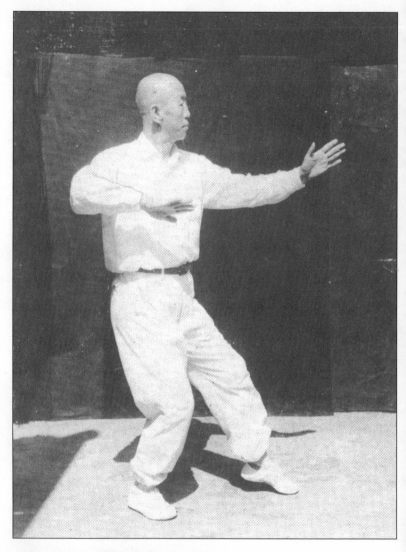

5. BRUSH KNEE AND TWIST STEP

摟膝拗步　　Lou Hsih Au Pu

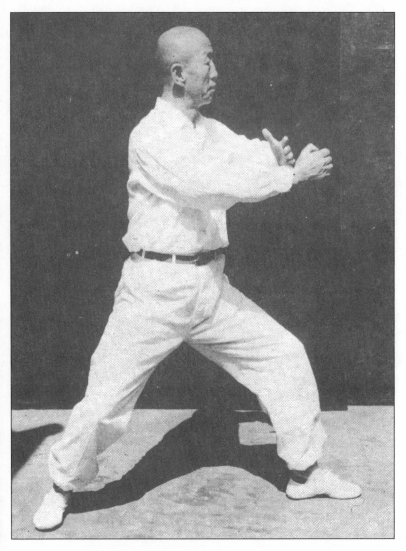

6. DEFLECT DOWNWARD, PARRY, AND PUNCH

搬、攔、捶   Pan, Lan, Ch'ui

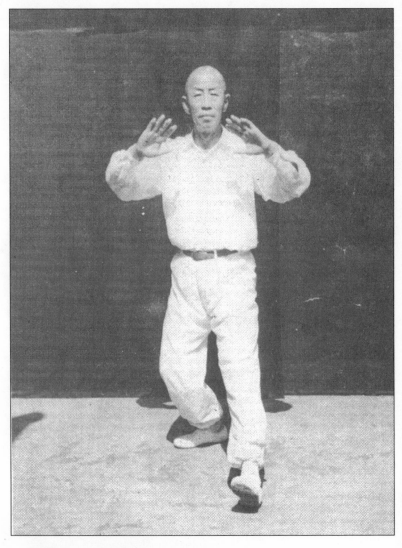

7. STEP UP, APPARENT CLOSE UP

上步、如封似開   Shang Pu, Ju Feng Shih Pi

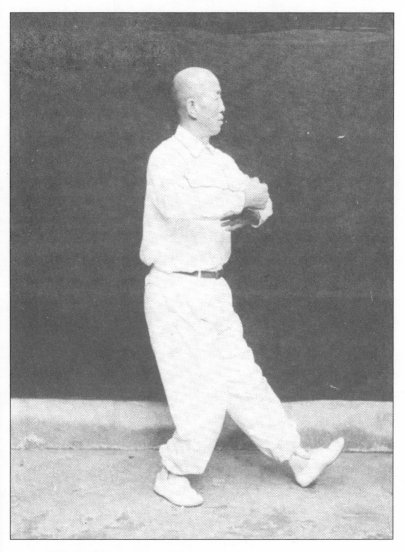

8. CARRY TIGER TO MOUNTAIN

抱虎歸山　　Pao Hu Kwei Shan

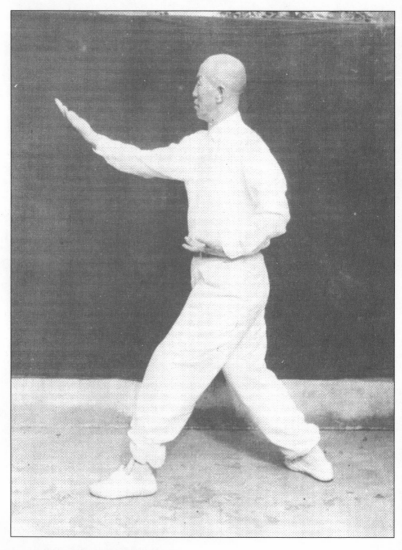

9. FIST UNDER ELBOW

肘底捶 Chou Ti Ch'ui

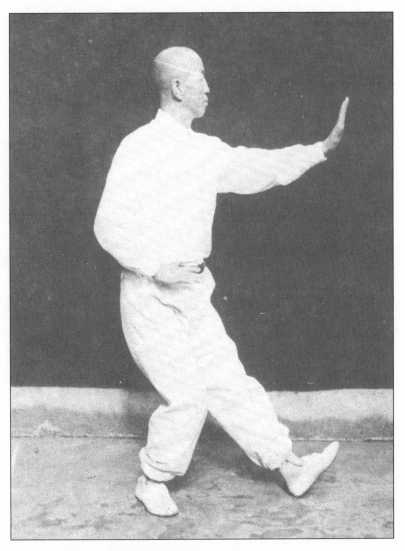

10. STEP BACK AND REPULSE MONKEY

倒攆猴　Tao Nien Hua

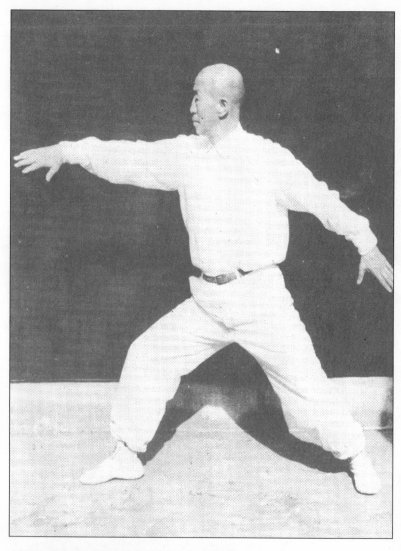

II. SLOW PALM SLANTING FLYING

挫掌斜飛　　Chao Chang Hsia Fei

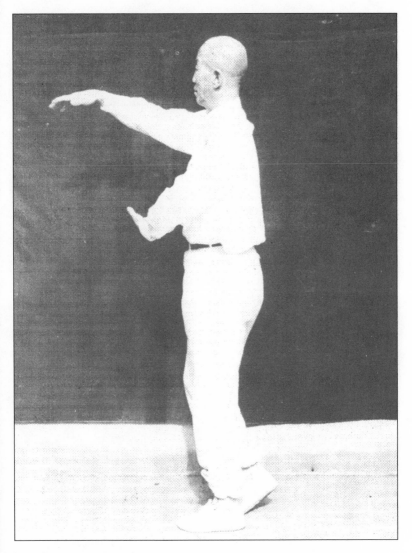

12. RAISE RIGHT HAND

右提手　Yu Ti Shou

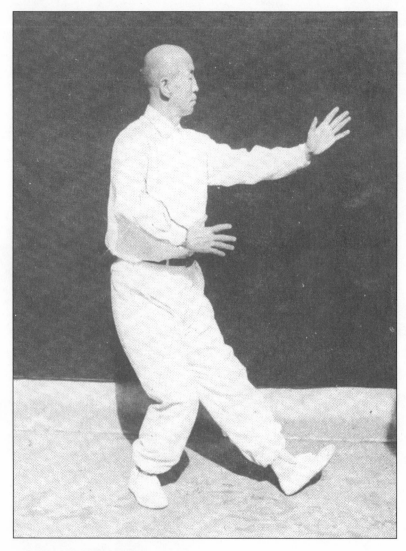

12. RAISE LEFT HAND

左提手　Tso Ti Shou

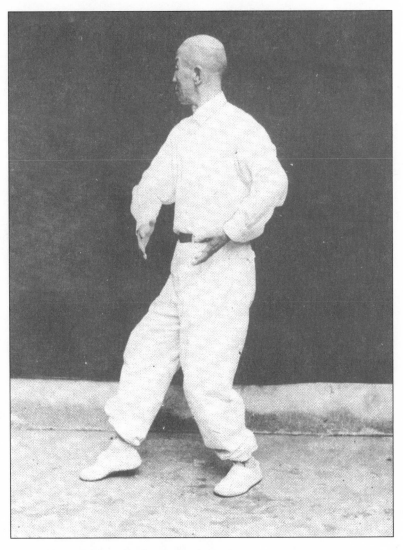

13. FLY PULLING BACK AND STEP UP

飛攦上勢　Fei Lu Shang Shih

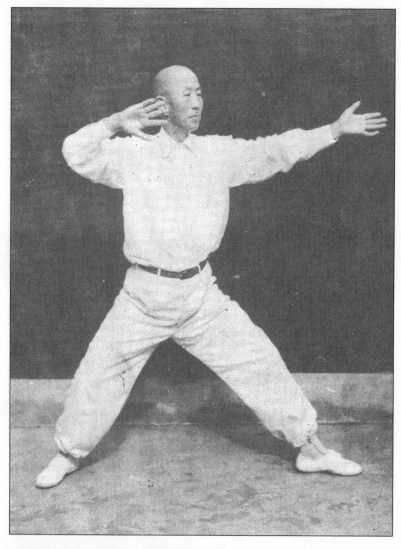

14. FAN THROUGH THE ARM

扇通臂　Shan Tung Pei

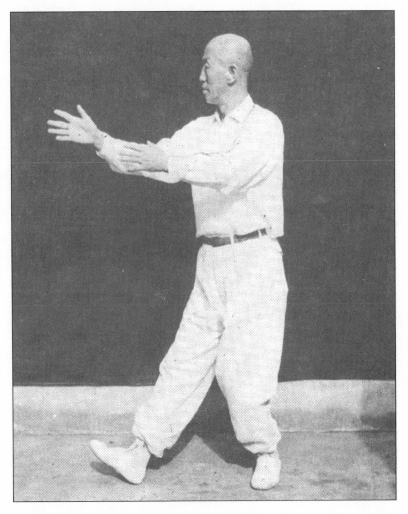

15. GREEN DRAGON DROPPING WATER

青龍出水　Chin Lung Cheu Hsiu

16. SINGLE WHIP

單鞭

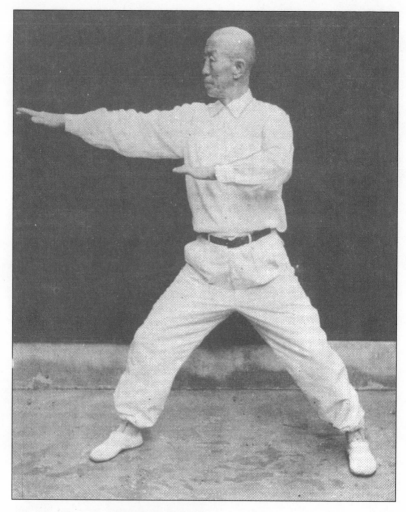

17. WAVE HANDS LIKE CLOUDS

雲 手 Yun Shou

18. SINGLE WHIP

單鞭

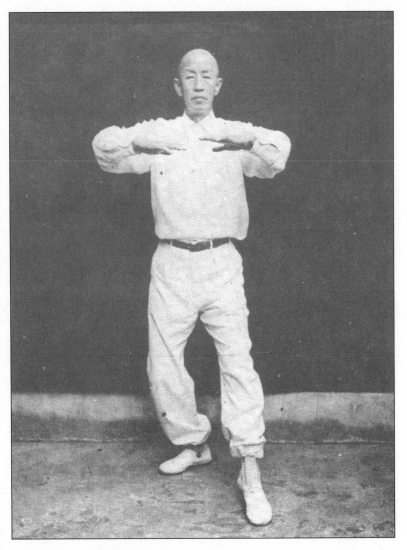

19. HIGH PAT ON HORSE

高探馬 Kao T'an Ma

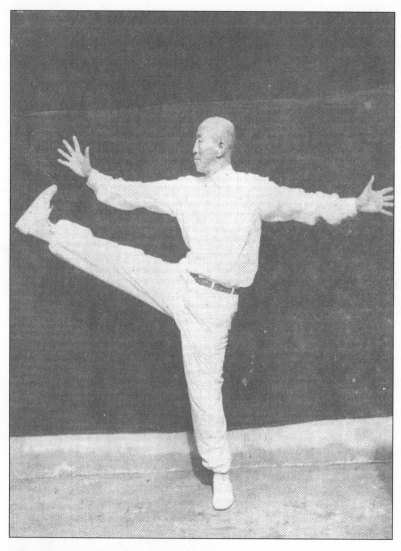

20. SEPARATION OF RIGHT FOOT

右 分 脚　Yu Fen Chiao

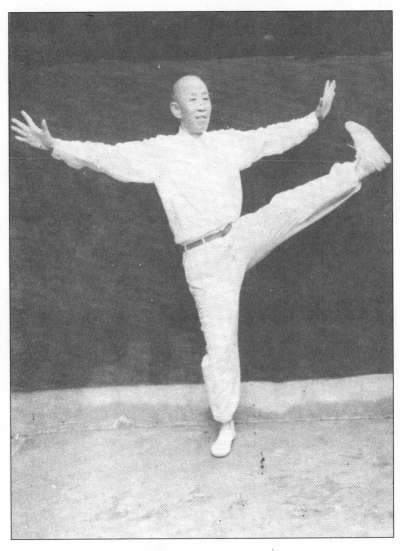

20. SEPARATION OF LEFT FOOT

左 分 脚 Tso Fen Chiao

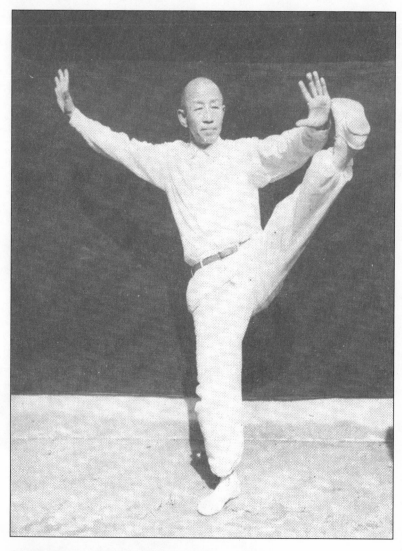

21. TURN AND KICK WITH SOLE

轉身蹬腳　Chuan Shen Teng Chiao

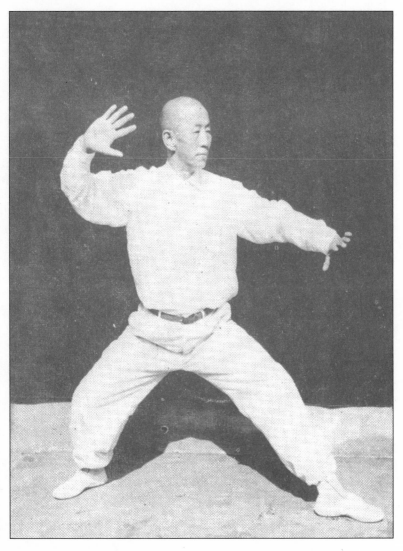

22. WIND BLOWING LOTUS LEAF (LEFT STYLE)

風擺荷葉（左式） Feng Pai Ho Yeh (Tso Shih)

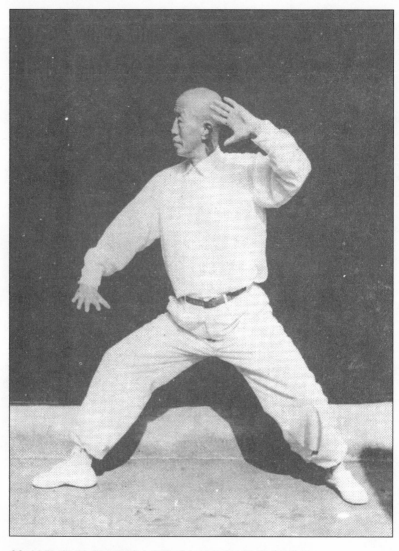

22. WIND BLOWING LOTUS LEAF (RIGHT STYLE)

風擺荷葉（右式） Feng Pai Ho Yeh (Yu Shih)

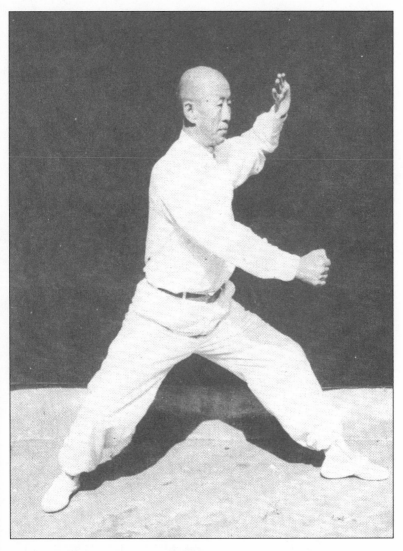

23. FINGER BLOCK UP WITH FIST

指 擋 捶　Shih Tang Ch'ui

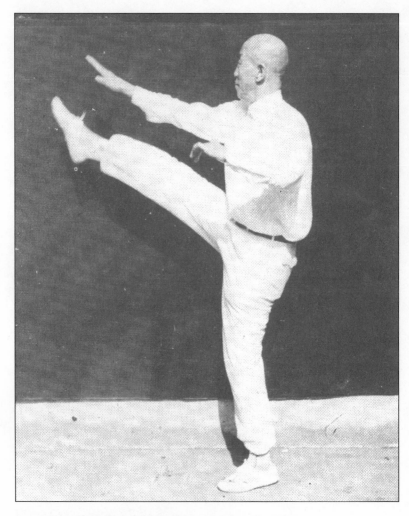

24. TURN ROUND KICKS TWO FEET UPWARD

翻身二起脚　　Fan Shen Er Shih Chiao

25. STEP UP, PARRY, AND PUNCH

上步搬攔捶

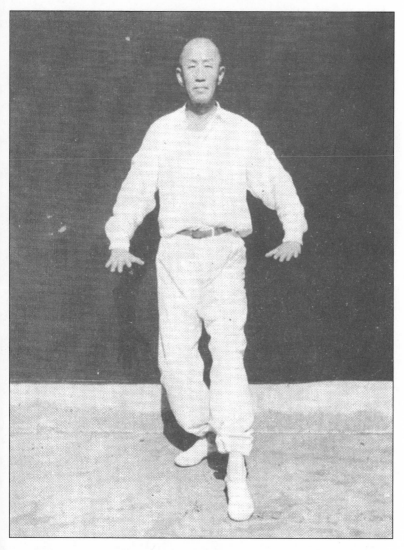

26. STEP BACK WITH ARMS BESIDE BODY

退步臂身　T'i Pu Bea Shen

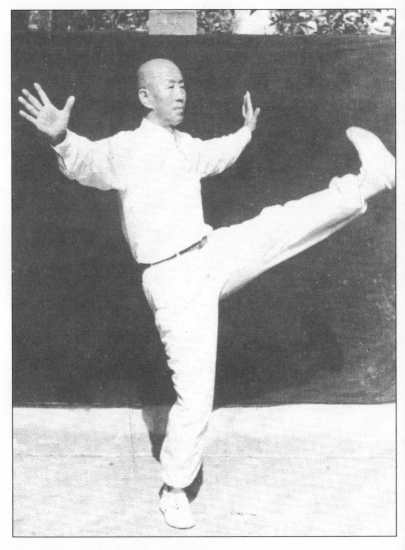

27. LEFT FOOT KICKS UP FORWARD

迎面踢脚 Yin Mean T'i Chiao

28. TURN AND KICK WITH SOLE

轉身蹬脚

29. STEP UP, PARRY, AND PUNCH

上步搬攔捶

30. APPARENT CLOSE-UP

如封似閉

31. CARRY TIGER TO THE MOUNTAIN

抱虎歸山

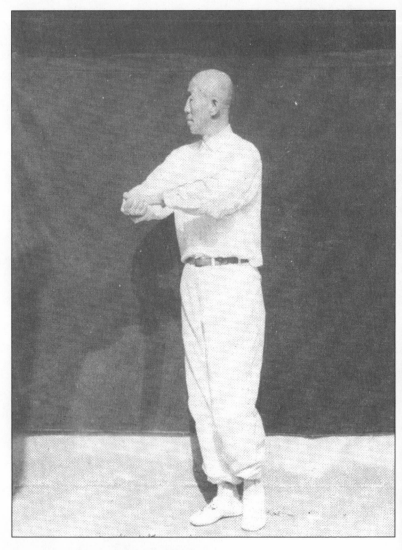

32. CHOP OPPONENT WITH FIST

撇身捶　Pi Shen Ch'ui

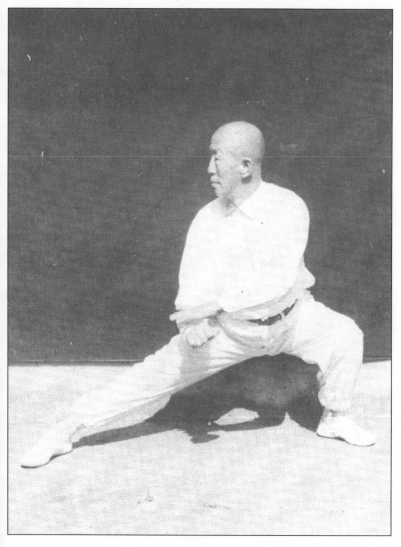

32. CHOP OPPONENT WITH FIST AND STEP DOWN

撇身捶下勢　Pi Shen Ch'ui Hsia Shih

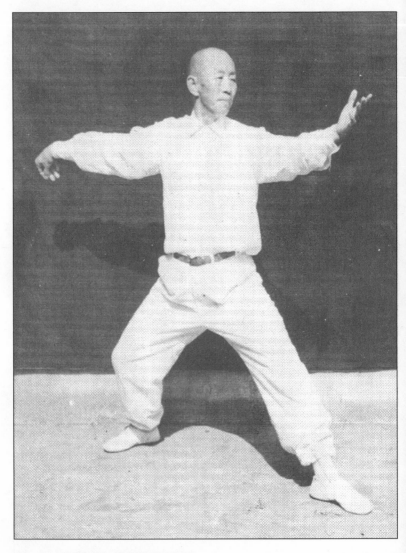

33. DIAGONAL SINGLE WHIP

斜單鞭　Hsia Tan Pien

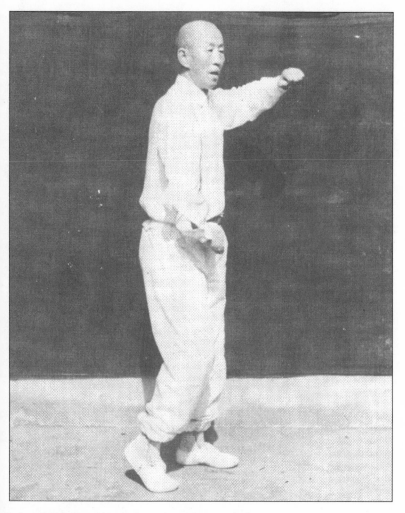

34. PARTITION OF WILD HORSE'S MANE

野馬分鬃　Yeh Ma Fen Tsung

35. DIAGONAL SINGLE WHIP

斜單鞭

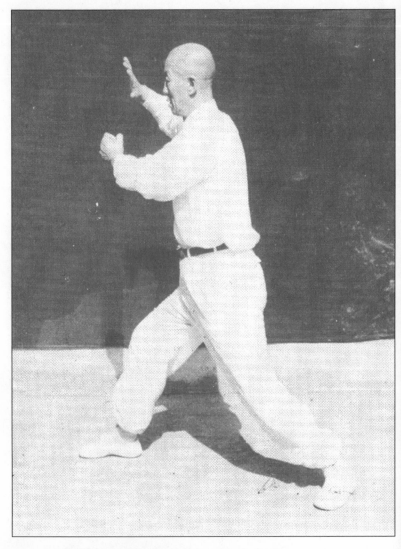

36. WORKING AT SHUTTLES INSIDE CLOUDS

雲裡穿梭 〔二〕　Yu-Li Chuan Shu (2)

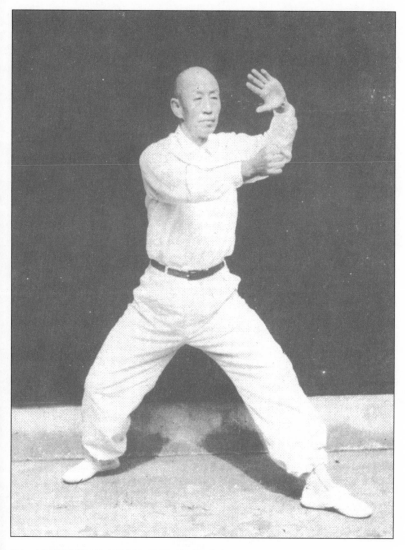

36. WORKING AT SHUTTLES INSIDE CLOUDS

雲裡穿梭 〔二〕 Yu-Li Chuan Shu (2)

37. STEP UP, GRASP BIRD'S TAIL

轉身攬雀尾

38. SINGLE WHIP

單鞭

39. WAVE HANDS LIKE CLOUDS

雲 手

40 SINGLE WHIP LOWERING DOWN

單鞭下勢

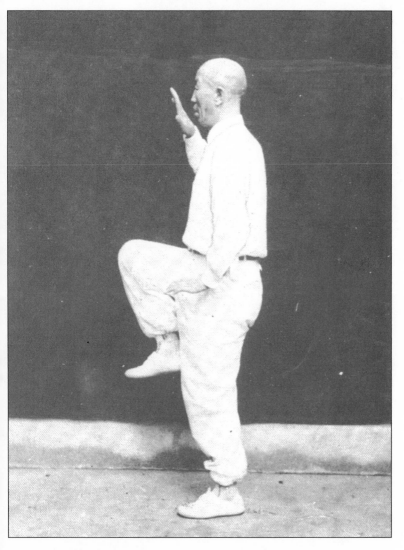

41. GOLDEN COCK STANDS ON ONE LEG

金鷄獨立　　Chin chi Tu Li

42. STEP BACK, REPULSE MONKEY

倒撵猴

43. SLOW PALM, SLANTING FLYING

挫掌斜飛

44. RAISE RIGHT HAND, RAISE LEFT HAND

右提手　左提手

45. FLY PULLING BACK AND STEP UP

飛撅上勢

46. FAN THROUGH THE ARM

扇通臂

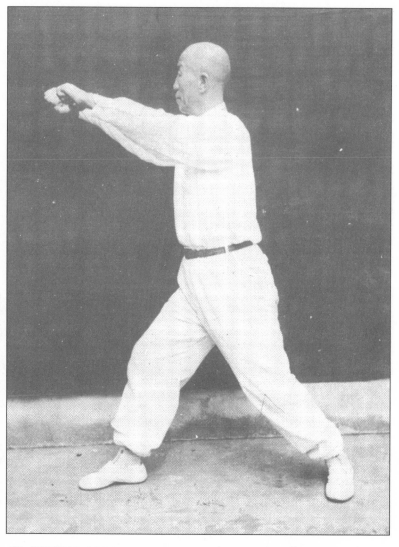

47. STRIKES OPPONENT'S EARS WITH BOTH FISTS

雙風貫耳　　Shuang Feng Kuan Er

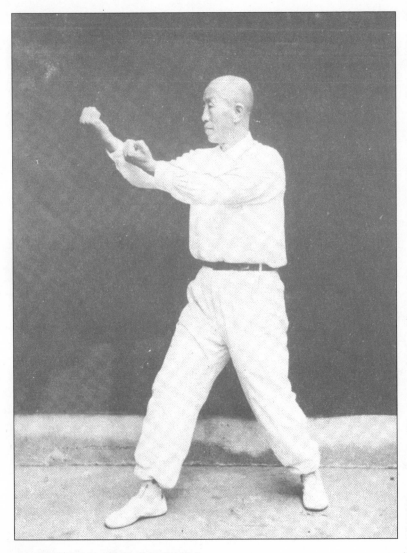

48. THROUGH SKY CANNON

通天砲　Tung Tien Pao

49. SINGLE WHIP

單鞭

50. WAVE HANDS LIKE CLOUDS

雲 手

51. SINGLE WHIP

單鞭

52. HIGH PAT ON HORSE

高探馬

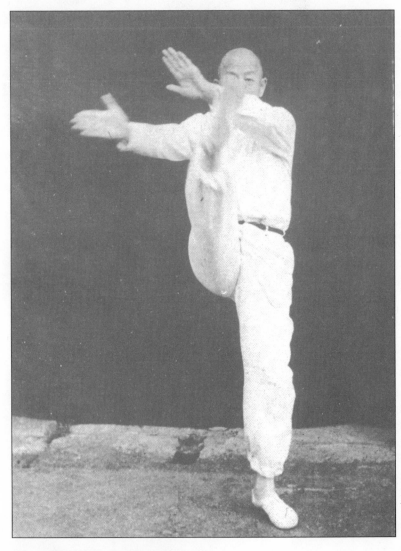

53. CROSS WAVE OF WATER LILY

十字擺蓮　Shih Tze Pai Lien

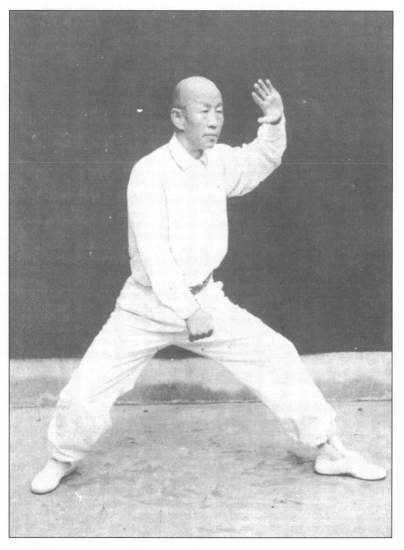

54. DOWNWARD FIST

栽　捶　Gei Ch'ui

55. STEP UP, GRASP BIRD'S TAIL

轉身攬雀尾

56. SINGLE WHIP

單鞭

57. WAVE HANDS LIKE CLOUDS

雲　手

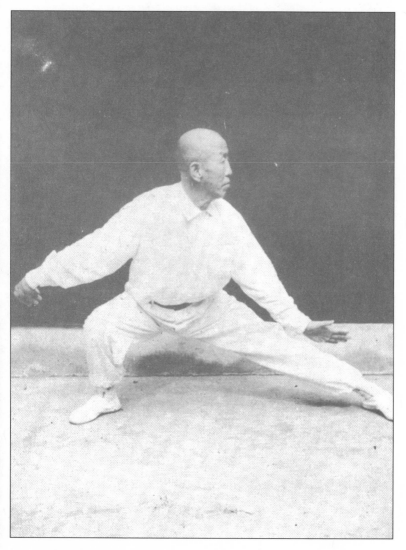

58. SINGLE WHIP DOWN

單鞭下勢　　Tan Pien Hsia Shih

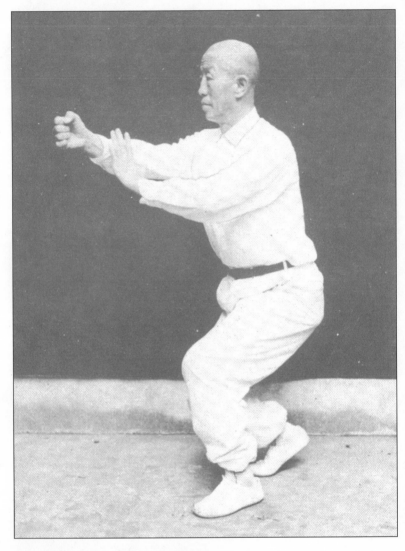

59. STEP UP TO FORM SEVEN STARS

上步七星　　Shan Pu Chi Hsing

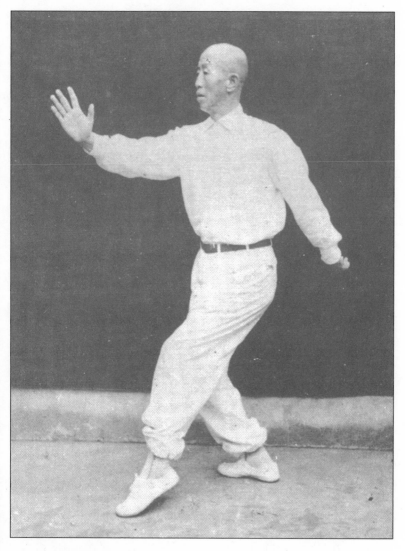

60. RETREAT TO RIDE TIGER

退步跨虎　　T'ui Pu K'ua Hu

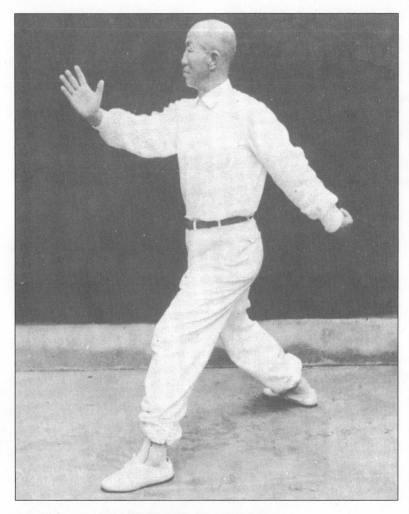

61. SLANTING BODY AND TURN THE MOON

斜身扭月　　Hsia Shen Neu Yea

62. WAVE LOTUS FOOT

擺 蓮 脚

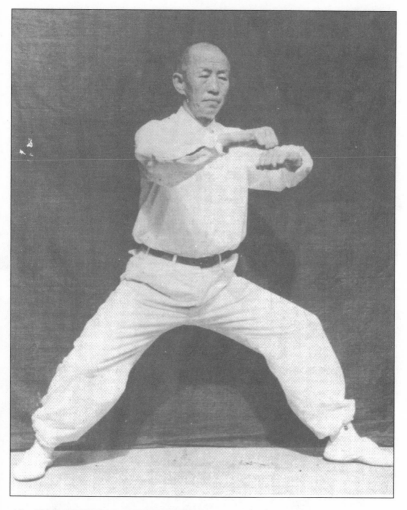

63. SHOOT TIGER WITH BOW

彎弓射虎　　Wan Kang She Hu

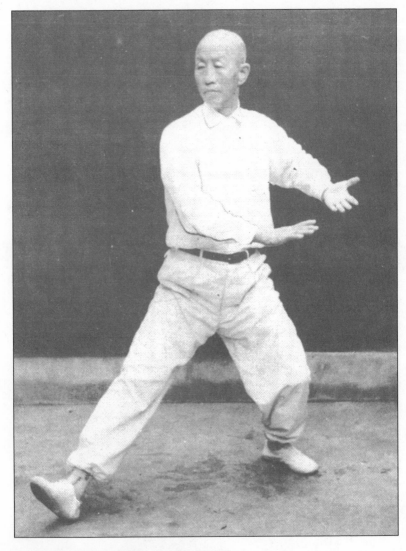

64. GRASP BIRD'S TAIL (LEFT STYLE)

左右攬雀尾　Tso Yu Lan Ch'iao Wei (Tso Shih)

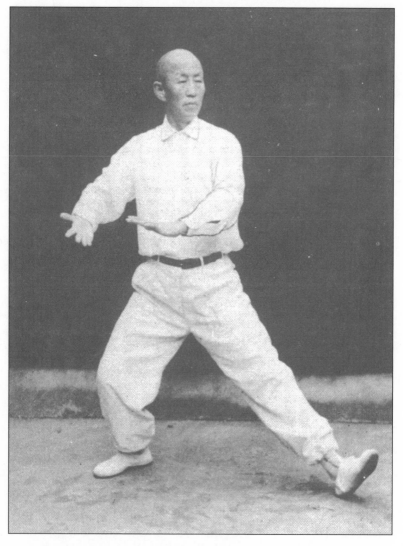

64. GRASP BIRD'S TAIL (RIGHT STYLE)

左右攬雀尾　Tso Yu Lan Ch'iao Wei (Yu Shih)

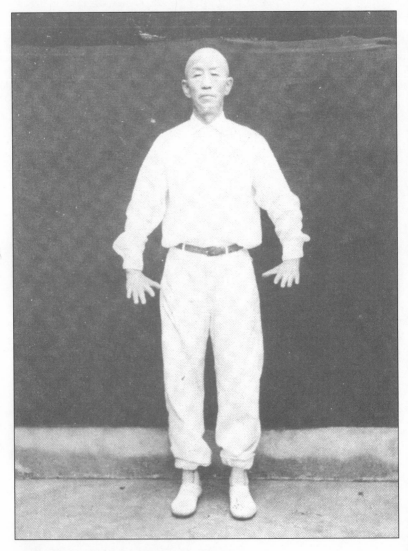

CONCLUSION OF GRAND TERMINUS

合 太 極　　He T'ai Chi

CHAPTER 8

Yu Chou Chuang
Universal Post

宇宙樁

Master Kuo Lien-Ying of martial arts (郭連蔭老師) was an expert of Tai-Chi Chuan (太極拳) and cultivated the most essential kungfu of this branch of martial arts, i.e. the Yu Chou Chuang.

This unusual exercise helps you to develop your mental health which gradually promotes your physical strength. It is especially useful for those who are engaged in office work and not familiar with manual labor.

When Master Kuo is doing this exercise, he gives you an image of immense potentiality, looking out into infinite space, with his monolithic figure in complete equilibrium both mentally and physically.

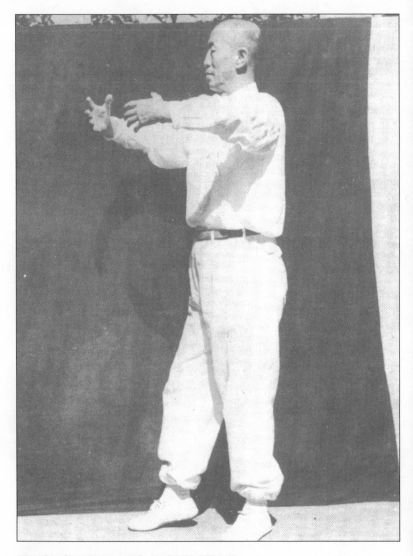

YU CHOU CHUANG (RIGHT STYLE)

宇宙樁（右式） Universal Post (Yu Chu Tsung) (Yu Shih)

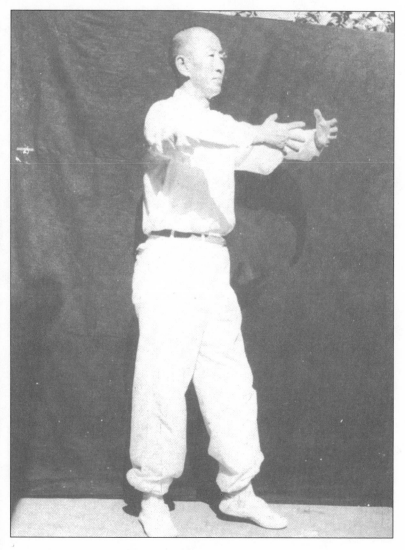

UNIVERSAL POST (LEFT STYLE)

宇宙樁（左式） (Yu Chu Tsung) (Tso Shih)

宇宙樁

宇宙樁功太奇特
大用外腓神素實
超以象外無隔彎不屈
大方太空俱適往
橫覽長風怛恬逸
寥寥遠瞻傲世外
昂首出銀乘返月
如鉛無束亦無我
無拘投水波紋線
如石意識內向抱
剎那上縱來兩膝
斷續屹立恒鍊冶
平明可守操縱得
可攻自求多福天行健
不可思議健身術

微妙玄通不可識
處處鬆開莫用力
返虛入渾勻氣息
圓圓融融任自然
窅然空縱凌雲筆
瀟洒脫一若為天下式
抱古鏡照神見道心
如入飄渺展矯翼
無限擴展無限大
乾坤萬象羅胸臆
一撐一抱無停止
積健為雄郤百疾
堅定信念最重要
五臟滋養自增殖

虛懷拱抱強為容
走雲連風御八極
不執不有空所空
氣流四肢無阻抑
荒荒油雲休天鈞
神態舒適守靜默
空潭瀉春素儲潔
如淥滿酒恍有物
漣漪盪漾向天際
若欲撐破宇宙殼
兩內腳眼往外撐
雜念屏除驅迷惑
淄磷不舍得環中
充沛活力惟此則
萬古難窺金丹訣

PILLAR OF THE UNIVERSE

the splendor of the universe is amazing
its mystery unfathomable
embracing all greatness effortlessly

its usefulness spreads to all ways,
expanding without effort
like the clouds and winds roaming in all directions

it transcends the reality of our world
balancing the spirit from out of emptiness
not insisting, not possessing, not caring
   for all worldliness

flexible, broad-minded, yet invincible
living smoothly and easily — one with nature
his ways are without contradiction

his works are smooth and easy
like brushes gliding among clouds
like swirling clouds in the sky

sweetly, the soothing wind roams alone
majestic and gentle
its attitudes are comfort and tranquillity

its loftiness is above all worldly phenomena
yet he holds the secret of the universe
its purity and chasteness are like the dawning of spring

as a lead-like silvery moon sailing by
it reflects from the ancient mirror
   the true heart of holiness
as a pure wine shows its clarity

uninhibited, selfless
as if rising above with wings to fly
higher and higher into the sky

like pool ripples from a thrown pebble
it expands boundlessly
as if to encompass the universe

be willing to embrace its ways
expand your chest like thousands of elephants
kick up your heels

follow up with high kicking knees
push with palm, persevere in practice
eliminate all distraction

the emperor shall establish
   lasting peace with just laws
health shall gather to heal a hundred ills
they shall not enter your sphere

its skill comprises both offense and defense
it is essential not to waver in your faith
fill yourself with power and energy

pray for the blessing of heavenly health
your five-organ system will flourish naturally
a thousand years of treasure secrets are locked here

better not to hesitate in practice[7]

FOR ARMS

To do this exercise, take the arrow stance with the left foot in front and the right foot in back. Place the left hand on the left side waist. Rotate the right arm from right shoulder, cross the left shoulder, over the left knee and repeat. (Don't overextend the arm back past the shoulder and keep your fingers straight). Repeat this motion 12 times. Then repeat the exercise in a reverse motion (rotate the right arm from right shoulder, over the left knee, and then cross the left shoulder).

Repeat the whole exercise for the left arm.

The Arm Rotation Exercise promotes relaxation of the shoulders, neck and chest. It also helps to improve breathing, reduce stress, and reduce feelings of anger. Students, computer operators and others can benefit from this exercise.

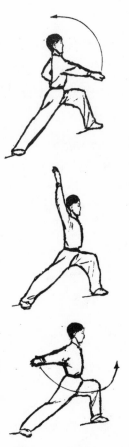

CHAPTER 9

I-Ching and the
Origins of Tai-Chi Philosophy

●

I consider myself most fortunate to have been married and lived with Sifu for more than 20 years. Sifu was a true master who practiced and taught Tai-Chi Chuan in the spirit of wholeness. The fabric of our everyday life was all part of my education. He encouraged me to study the traditional philosophy of China and to weave its principles into my life and practice.

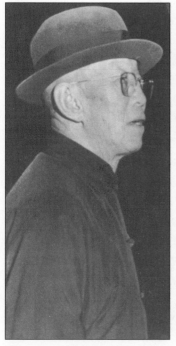

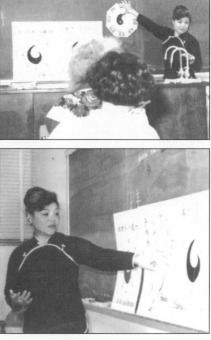

The image of Sifu is great encouragement for teaching.

My appreciation for Sifu's teaching, San Francisco State University, 1980.

Since Sifu's passing, I have made a series of journeys to China in order to research the roots of traditional Tai-Chi philosophy; for it is from

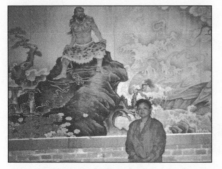

these roots that Tai-Chi Chuan —like all of the treasured arts and sciences of China—developed and flourished. It is my sincere hope that this work will encourage later generations to pursue further research. In doing so the student can gradu-

Simmone Kuo with mural of Fu Xi observing nature from atop the mountain, 1993.

ally reach a deeper contemplation of the source.

The most ancient and fundamental expression of Tai-Chi philosophy is the *I-Ching* which studies the dynamic process through which the forms of our world are created, sustained and destroyed. The origins of this knowledge are pre-historical, more than 5000 years old. Fu-Xi, the legendary first emperor of China, and founder of the Shang dynasty, is revered as the one who brought Tai-Chi philosophy into Chinese culture.

Fu-Xi envisioned the cosmos as an ongoing process of change, in which phenomena arise from and return to the void. He observed the waxing and waning of light, the cycling of the seasons and the revolutions of the celestial bodies. Understanding that the same dynamic laws govern every level of creation, he envisioned the whole world as the interplay of the primordial yin and yang energies. All

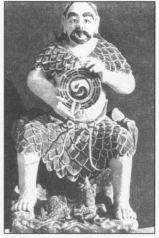

Fu-Xi (c. 2800 B.C.E.)

伏　羲

史料記載，「三皇」伏羲、神衣、軒猿、是人類始祖，特別是伏羲。他智慧超人與眾不同。他經常留意觀察分析研究各種目遊現象，發明了燒，炙巢養教會人们飲食的習慣並利用光影創造了陰陽、四象、五形、八卦這一套符号，幫助人们認識自遊災害發生的部份規律和避開違自然災害的危害。世界人類的「開天明道」都是伏羲的功德和貢献。

of the universe is the unfolding of a single event, and all creatures are transient forms, each a unique and shifting blend of yin and yang, essence and substance. The union of yin and yang, which is called Tai-Chi, gives birth to this world and all its possible forms.

A fundamental principle of Tai-Chi philosophy is that none of the 10000 things is pure yin or pure yang: each is an embodiment of Tai-Chi. Therefore the traditional symbol for Tai-Chi shows the presence of yin within yang and yang within yin.

Fu-Xi's own notation forms the basis for the *I-Ching*: yin is represented as a broken line and yang as an unbroken one. When these two are taken three at a time, there are eight possibilities and these are the eight trigrams or Pa Kua.

In this diagram, white dots are yang, black dots yin.

When these eight trigrams are taken two at a time, there are 64 possibilities and these are the sixty-four hexagrams of the *I-Ching*, which may be understood as 64 archetypal situations or fundamental configu-

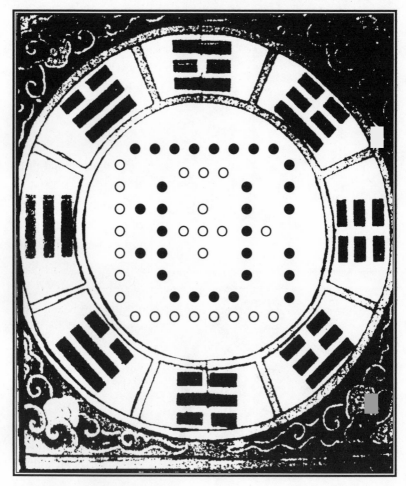

Ceiling painting of Pa-Kua diagram

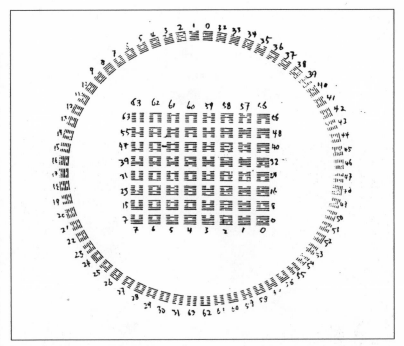

Image of the circle of 64 hexagrams

rations of energy. Tai-Chi philosophy inquires into the dynamics through which the hexagrams are related to one another, and how they are transformed into each other through the interplay of their yin and yang components.

Although we generally know the *I-Ching* as a book, in its purest form, the *I-Ching* consists simply of the graphic representations of the 64 hexagrams.

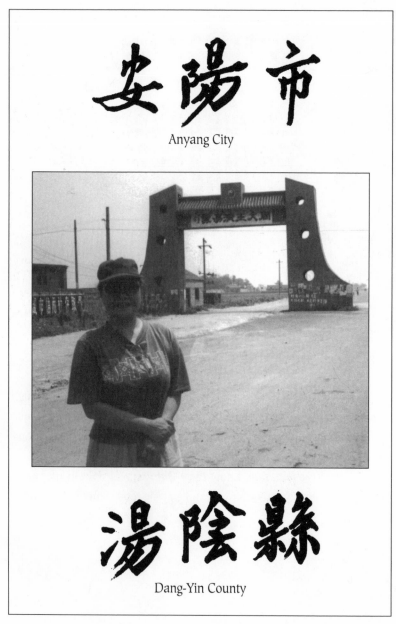

安陽市

Anyang City

湯陰縣

Dang-Yin County

Simmone Kuo's visit to the second capital city of China, 1997

The most ancient existing commentaries to the *I-Ching* are those of King Wen and his son, the Duke of Chou, the founders of China's second major dynasty. The Chou dynasty followed the Shang and flourished for several centuries from 1100 B.C.E. to 700 B.C.E.

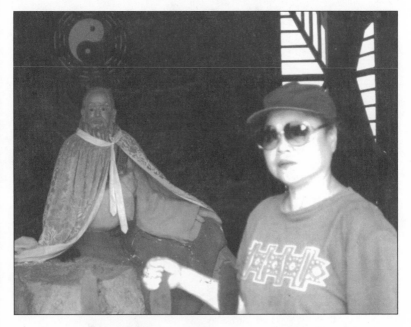

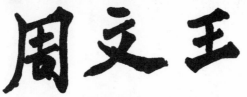

Chou Wen-Wang

周易概說

上古時期，隨着生產活动的发展，人们開始發现自然界的一些规律，尤其是在事物发生发展中起决定作用的两种对立因素，以为逆四种立相滑長缺一不可的因素是任何事物都具有并且固有的屬性。後来人们將其中一方称「陰」另一方称「陽」，開始形成中國文化特有的「陰」「陽」思念。

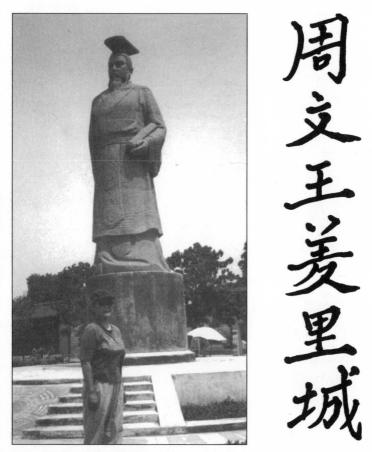

周文王姜里城

Statue of Chou Wen-Wang

Chou Wen-Wang (posthumously designated King Wen by his son) lived in the time of upheaval between the Shang and Chou dynasties. During eight years of imprisonment in his 80s, the elderly Wen had ample opportunity to reflect upon his life experiences and to contemplate the nature of the world. He created the first comprehensive commentaries on the *I-Ching*. These include the "judgement" for each hexagram, together with line by line commentaries for each of its six lines.

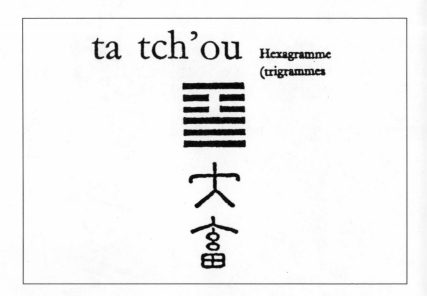

Ta shows a man stretching out his arms and means great.

In *Tch'ou* one sees from bottom to top: a field which produces a plant fibre — placed on a distaff and hanging from a roof. This is the image of acquired knowledge, of education.

Ta Tch'ou is thus education in what is great.

Judgement: A great education gives one self-confidence and draws one toward perfection.

Development:

1. In the face of danger, it is better to break off than to seek to conquer by force.

2. When the carriage is in difficulty . . .

3. There will not be an accident if the horses are well trained.

4. The yoke is the only way to train an ox for work in the fields.

5. A castrated wild-boar has only inoffensive defenses.

6. The sky is vast, and takes a long time to traverse.[8]

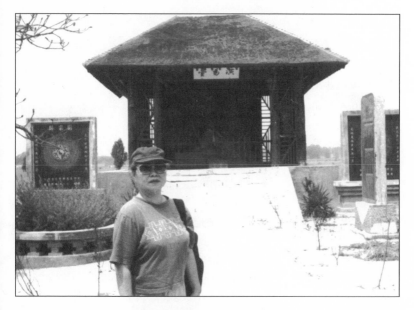

安陽市 , 湯蔭縣

The site of Chou's imprisonment

The primary use of the *I-Ching* is as a focus for contemplation and an instrument for inquiry. Given its ingenious conception and universal scope, the *I-Ching* can assist in the investigation of any sort of situation: what forces are currently at play, how the situation may develop, etc. Indeed, the *I-Ching* has played a crucial role in the development of every important aspect of Chinese culture: clock, calendar, agriculture, craft, feng-shui, health practices, philosophy, relationships, social formation, historical cycles—all these have been influenced and shaped through the application of Tai-Chi philosophy. In this regard, Tai-Chi Chuan may be considered the system for self-defense and self-cultivation which has resulted from the application of Tai-Chi philosophy to the rich tradition of Chinese martial arts.

Over the centuries, then, successive layers of commentary and interpretation have arisen and attached themselves to the bare bones of the *I-Ching*. All of the most important philosophers of China—from Confucius to Chang San-Feng, the creator of Tai-Chi Chuan—have studied this classic of wisdom. Many have left fascinating commentaries. The Jewish Torah with its

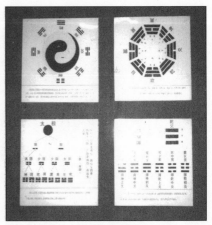

安陽市,湯陰縣

successive layers of commentary (Mishnah, Talmud, New Testament, Koran, etc.) is similar to the *I-Ching*, as a text of fundamental wisdom surrounded by successive generations of commentary and interpretation.

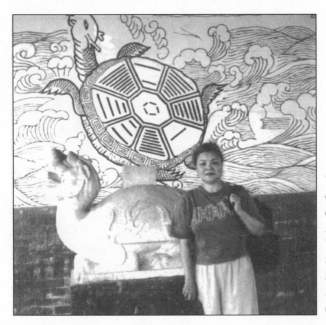

This image comes from a wall of Emperor Chou Temple. The turtle's shell bears a resemblance to the eight trigrams.

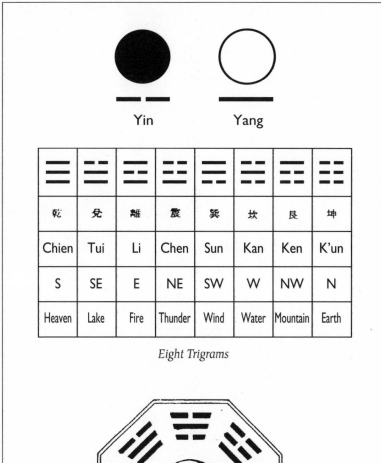

Yin   Yang

乾	兌	離	震	巽	坎	艮	坤
Chien	Tui	Li	Chen	Sun	Kan	Ken	K'un
S	SE	E	NE	SW	W	NW	N
Heaven	Lake	Fire	Thunder	Wind	Water	Mountain	Earth

Eight Trigrams

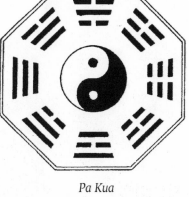

Pa Kua

CHAPTER 10

Supplementary Literature

●

THE SAYINGS OF
Lao Tzu

老　子

四
二
章

42

The Way begot one,
And the one, two;
Then the two begot three
And three, all else.

All things bear the shade on their backs
And the sun in their arms;
By the blending of breath
From the sun and the shade,
Equilibrium comes to the world.

Orphaned, or needy, or desolate, these
Are conditions much feared and disliked;
Yet in public address, the king
And the nobles account themselves thus.
So a loss sometimes benefits one
Or a benefit proves to be loss.

What others have taught
I also shall teach:
If a violent man does not come
To a violent death,
I shall choose him to teach me.[9]

道生一，一生二，二生三，三生萬物。

萬物負陰而抱陽，沖氣以爲和。

人之所惡，唯孤寡不穀，而侯王以爲稱。故物，或損之而益，或益之而損。

人之所教；我亦教之。强梁者，不得其死。吾將以爲教父。

THE SAYINGS OF
Lao Tzu

老 子

1

There are ways but the Way is
    uncharted;
There are names but not nature in
    words:
Nameless indeed is the source of
    creation
But things have a mother and she has
    a name

The secret waits for the insight
Of eyes unclouded by longing:
Those who are bound by desire
See only the outward container.

These two come paired but distinct
By their names.
Of all things profound,
Say that their pairing is deepest,
The gate to the root of the world.[10]

一 章

道可道，非常道；名可名，非常名。無，名天地之始；有，名萬物之母。

故常無欲，以觀其妙；常有欲，以觀其徼。

此兩者，同出而異名，同謂之玄。玄之又玄，衆妙之門。

唐诗三百首新译

English-Chinese
300 TANG POEMS
A New Translation

春曉

孟浩然

春眠不覺曉，
處處聞啼鳥。
夜來風雨聲，
花落知多少？

A Spring Morning

This morn of spring in bed I'm lying,
Not woke up till I hear birds crying.
After one night of wind and showers,
How many are the fallen flowers![11]

—Meng Haoran

唐诗三百首新译

English-Chinese
300 TANG POEMS
A New Translation

楓橋夜泊　　張繼

月落烏啼霜滿天，
江楓漁火對愁眠。
姑蘇城外寒山寺，
夜半鐘聲到客船。

Mooring at Night by Maple Bridge

The moon goes down, crows cry under the frosty sky,
Dimly-lit fishing boats 'neath maples sadly lie.
Beyond the Gusu walls the Temple of Cold Hill
Rings bells which reach my boat, breaking the midnight still.[12]

—Zhang Ji

古柏行　杜甫

孔明廟前有老柏，柯如青銅根如石。霜皮溜雨四十圍，
黛色參天二千尺。雲來氣接巫峽長，月出寒通雪山白。
君臣已與時際會，樹木猶爲人愛惜。憶昨路遶錦亭東，
先主武侯同閟宮。崔嵬枝幹郊原古，窈窕丹青戶牖空。
落落盤據雖得地，冥冥孤高多烈風。扶持自是神明力，
正直原因造化功。大廈如傾要梁棟，萬牛迴首邱山重！
不露文章世已驚，未辭剪伐誰能送？苦心豈免容螻蟻，
香葉終經宿鸞鳳。志士幽人莫怨嗟，古來材大難爲用！

1.

唐诗三百首新译

English-Chinese
300 TANG POEMS
A New Translation

The Ancient Cypress

There is an ancient cypress in front of the Kongming Fane*,
With branches bronzy and roots seemingly of stony cane.
The smooth and hoary trunk is thick for forty arms to span around,
Its dark green leaves wave in the sky two thousand feet beyond.
The Emperor and his premier had met in a juncture of times,
The visitors now treasure still the arbour in its prime.
The clouds bring its imposing airs to the Wu Gorge's gloom;
The moon reflects its coldness to the Snow Mountain's white dome.
I remember east of the Jin Jiang Pavilion the path.

To a fane where Liu Bei and Kongming are shrined in the
    same garden.
The giant trees there clothed the outfields in an archaic shade;
The doors opened to the hollow halls with pictures dimly made.

Though independently this plant has had its blessed place,

Yet the mountain squalls shake the lonely highness without grace.

It is the deities who support it standing high and neat,

And the upright manner is due to the Creator's feat.

If a great mansion is on the tilt, it needs a ridgepole,

Thousands of cattle would look back since the tree they couldn't
pull.

The people praise the potential sap within the plain mould,

It would fain be cut down, yet who may carry it to the world?

The bitter core of it did not prevent the ants to bore;

The phoenix yet came among the sweet leaves as a nest in store.

Let not the ambitious complain that they are abused,

For from old, all rare material is seldom justly used![13]

—Du Fu

*Kongming, courtesy name of Zhuge Liang, a hero of the 3 Kings Dynasty.
In memory of him, more than one fane was built after his death.*

CHINA'S GREAT CLASSIC
THE SAYINGS OF
MENCIUS

Poor, rich,
failure, success

Keep your integrity
don't leave the Way[14]

窮不失義

達不離道

孟子七卷
三頁

The Sayings of CONFUCIUS

論語

一 學而篇

1 子曰：「學而時習之，不亦說乎？有朋自遠方來，不亦樂乎？人不知而不慍，不亦君子乎？」

2 有子曰：「其為人也孝弟，而好犯上者鮮矣！不好犯上，而好作亂者，未之有也。君子務本，本立而道生。孝弟也者，其為人之本與！」

3 子曰：「巧言、令色，鮮矣仁！」

4 曾子曰：「吾日三省吾身：為人謀，而不忠乎？與朋友交，而不信乎？傳不習乎？」

THE SAYINGS OF
CONFUCIUS

Chapter I

As one learns . . .

1

"How pleasant it is to repeat constantly what we are learning!

"How happy we are when some friend returns from a long trip!

"To remain unconcerned though others do not know of us — that is to be Great Man!"

2

Yu Jo has said, "The filial and fraternal who are fond of offending their superiors are indeed few. Those who bring confusion to our midst always begin by being fond of offending their superiors.

"Great Man applies himself to the fundamentals, for once the fundamentals are there System comes into being. It is filial duty and fraternal duty that are fundamental to Manhood-at-its-best."

3

"Clever talk and a domineering manner have little to do with being man-at-his-best."

4

Tseng Ts'an once said, "Daily I examine myself on three points: Have I failed to be loyal in my work for others? Have I been false with my friends? Have I failed to pass on that which I was taught?"[15]

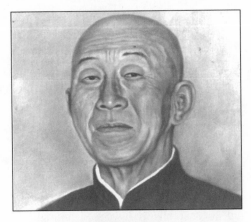

郭連蔭
Kuo Lien-Ying

郭 盧 瀅 如
Simmone L. Kuo
(Lu Ying-Ru)

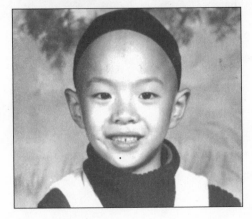

郭 中 美
Kuo Chung-Mei

Notes

1. Pu Rey, the brother of the last Emperor of China, wrote this poem for Kuo Lien-Ying's *Tai-Chi Chuan Rhythm*. Translation by Simu Kuo and Jeffrey Kessler.

2. All references to the I-Ching can be found in the Wilhelm/Baynes translation: *The I-Ching or Book of Changes*, Princeton University Press, Princeton, 1977.

3. Von Franz, Marie-Louise, *Puer Aeternus*, Sigo Press, Santa Monica, 1981, p. 5-7.

4. Frankl, Viktor, *Man's Search for Meaning: An Introduction to Logotherapy*, Beacon Press, Boston, 1962, pp. 124-126.

5. Illich, Ivan, *Medical Nemesis, The Expropriation of Health*, Random House, New York, 1976, pp. 168-169.

6. For further information, see Kuo, Simmone, *Long Life, Good Health through Tai-Chi Chuan*.

7. Poem translated by Jeffrey Chang and Jeffrey Kessler.

8. Lavier, J., *Le Livre de la Terre et du Ciel*, Editions Tchou, Paris, 1973, p. 87.

9. Lao Tzu, *The Sayings of Lao-Tzu*, trans. By Blakney, R. B., Confucius Publishing Co., Taipei, 1959, p. 84.

10. *op. cit.*, p. 2.

11. *300 Tang Poems*, trans. by Xu Yuan-Zhong, China Translation Export Co., Beijing, 1987, p. 28.

12. *op. cit.*, trans. Xu Yuan-Zhong, p. 224.

13. *op. cit.*, trans. Wu Juntao, p. 178.

14. Mencius, *The Works of Mencius* from *The Four Books*, trans. by Legge, James, Oxford University Press, Oxford, 1892, p. 453.

15. Confucius, *The Sayings of Confucius*, trans. by Ware, James, Confucius Publishing Co., Taipei, 1958, p. 2.

Caligraphy on pages 99 and 104 done by Rosita Young.